Contents

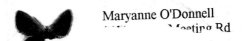
GUESS WHAT CAME TO DINNER

PARASITES AND YOUR HEALTH

Ann Louise Gittleman

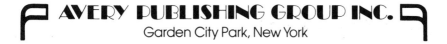
AVERY PUBLISHING GROUP INC.
Garden City Park, New York

The procedures in this book are based upon the research, personal and professional experience of the author. Should the reader have any questions regarding the appropriateness of any procedure or material mentioned, the publisher and author strongly suggest consulting a professional health-care advisor.

Because any material or procedure can be misused, the author and publisher are not responsible for any adverse effects or consequences resulting from the use of any of the preparations, materials, or procedures suggested in this book. However, the publisher believes that this information should be available to the public.

Cover design: Ann Vestal
Cover photo: J. Michael Dombroski
In-house editor: Linda Comac
Typesetter: Bonnie Fried

Library of Congress Cataloging-in-Publication Data

Gittleman, Ann Louise
    Guess what came to dinner : parasites and your health / by Ann Louise Gittleman.
        p. cm.
    Includes bibliographical references and index.
    ISBN 0-89529-570-9 (pbk.) : $9.95
    1. Parasitic diseases—Popular works. I. Title.
RC119.G58 1993   93-15449
616.9'6—d   CIP

Printed in the United States of America.

10 9 8 7 6 5 4 3 2 1

This book is dedicated to
Hazel R. Parcells, Ph.D., D.C., N.D.,
whose relentless search for truth
and the underlying causes of disease
inspired my life's work in the science of nutrition.

Acknowledgments

I gratefully acknowledge the pioneering work of researchers Dr. LuCrece Dowell, Dr. Hermann Bueno, Dr. Louis Parrish, Dr. Leo Litter, Dr. Peter Weina, Dr. Leo Galland, and Dr. Martin Wolfe. Thanks also to the natural healers among us who have recognized parasites as a primary cause of human disease, the Reverend Hanna Kroeger, Dr. Fred Houston, and Ann Wigmore.

There are several doctors with whom I have had contact over the years about my experience and research in parasites. Some of these health practitioners have always been aware of the problem of parasites, and others have gone on to include parasite testing in their practices. I salute Dr. Gary Ross, Dr. Abram Ber, Dr. Elson Haas, Dr. Zane Gard, Dr. Nate Mayfield, Dr. Warren Levin, and Andreas Marx, OMD. I salute health practitioners Lou Talento, Glenn Wilcox, and Angelique Cook-Wilcox. I especially acknowledge Dr. Shirley Scott, who has made parasitic disease a major focus of her practice.

Thanks also to Stuart Gittleman for his research assistance, to James Templeton for his insight and encouragement, to Rudy Shur and Linda Comac for their editorial guidance, and to Alice Q. Swanson for her invaluable support and expertise in making this book a reality.

Last but not least, to Bernie, for reasons only he knows.

Foreword

*P*arasites are the missing diagnosis in the genesis of
many chronic health problems, including diseases
of the gastrointestinal tract and endocrine system.
Most individuals would be truly amazed if they knew the
extraordinarily high number of Americans who are unknowingly infected by parasites acquired during world
travel or in the United States. Nutritionist Ann Louise
Gittleman has provided an invaluable public health service in writing a book about a subject that urgently requires
more medical attention and public awareness.

The impact of parasitic action is very broad, ranging
from what we may call a "localized infection" to one "at a
distance." In the former type, the parasitic activity produces
irritative, inflammatory, and/or mechanical problems such
as obstructions of hollow organs like the common bile ducts
and intestines. These conditions can usually be diagnosed

and treated by an experienced parasitologist or a specialist in tropical medicine. In the "at a distance" type, the parasites produce most intriguing and unexpected manifestations in systems that only recently have been discovered to be target organs for the parasite toxins.

It is of tremendous pragmatic importance to consider various syndromes as puzzling occurrences that result from the activities of several types of parasites in the human body. These syndromes include chronic fatigue, hypoglycemia, hypothyroidism, hypoadrenalism, dysgonadism (protein dysfunction in the genito-gonadal area), chronic upper respiratory tract ailments, depressive manifestations, depressed libido, and endometriosis.

To reach a positive diagnosis, it is imperative to utilize new technologies and to train experts in the field of parasitology. However, it is regretful that such technologies and training are far from realization and from a high level of scientific accuracy. There are still far too many non-believers preventing the march forward through the fascinating world of parasitic diseases.

The contribution of Ms. Gittleman, I do believe, is going to be very substantial and material to the general population's knowledge of the tremendous impact of parasite-related manifestations all over the world. The author's solid background in the area of nutrition is going to make this book highly ranked in the multidisciplinary arena of clinical parasitology.

Dr. Hermann R. Bueno
Fellow of Royal Society of Tropical Medicine
and Hygiene of London

Preface

*T*his book is purposefully designed to open up a can of worms. I know that the subject matter will not be the most pleasant reading material, but parasites are allowed to persist precisely because we revile the idea of housing worms.

The woman who typed the first draft of this book presented me with a copy of the manuscript and remarked, "You ruined my life!" She then proceeded to relate to me that thirty-one years ago, her infant son had been infected with pinworms. The manuscript had brought back all the feelings she had buried . . . repulsion at first discovering these little thread-like worms wiggling in her son's diaper . . . not wanting to touch her own baby . . . feelings of somehow being a "bad" mother. But she didn't ignore the situation, nor was she in denial. She sought help not only for her baby, but for her whole family, and instituted a periodic deworming for all the children throughout their childhood.

It is my hope in writing this book that once you realize the extent of the parasite epidemic in America today, you will react as did my typist and take the proper measures, from diagnosis, to treatment, to prevention. I suggest you take this book to your doctor so that he can also be informed about this emerging health crisis

The first part of the book will introduce you to the major reasons parasites are found in America today, what they are, how they do their damage, and how to recognize their symptoms and effects on the body. Then there will be discussions of the most common methods of transmission, from food and water to pets and day-care centers. The final chapters deal with ways to diagnosis, treat, and prevent parasites. A special parasite-risk questionnaire is included for you and your doctor. A glossary is provided to help you become familiar with the jargon, and the appendix provides drug information for your doctor.

I hope that after reading this book, you will come away with a greater understanding of how we all are at risk for parasites, and what each individual can do to reduce that risk.

My own interest in parasites goes back to 1974 when one of my nutrition mentors, Dr. Hazel Parcells, first made me aware that parasites could be a very real, and very prevalent, problem in mainstream America. Since that time, I have clipped, collected, written away for, and acquired enough information on worms to fill several filing cabinets.

In 1984, I was interviewed on the subject of parasites by a national health magazine. The enormous response to that interview brought many concerned individuals to my office. I have since been referring hundreds of people to doctors and laboratories for parasite testing, and my own practice has become overwhelmingly devoted to the nutritional implications of parasitic diseases.

Over the years, I have seen a multitude of patients with symptoms of chronic fatigue, hypoglycemia, food allergy, spastic colon, and respiratory disorders get well when parasites were eradicated from their systems. I feel that many individuals with unexplained health problems can benefit from a book of this kind.

Ann Louise Gittleman, M.S.

Introduction

D o you feel tired most of the time? Are you experiencing digestive problems—gas, bloating, constipation or diarrhea—that come and go but never really clear up? Do you suffer from food sensitivities and environmental intolerances? Have you developed allergic-like reactions and can't understand why? Are you depressed? Do you have difficulty gaining or losing weight no matter what you do? Have you even tried a yeast control program that helped to some degree but know you can't stay away from bread, alcohol, fruit, and fruit juices all your life? Do you sense something is not quite right with you but just can't figure out the cause—and, for that matter, neither can your doctor?

If these symptoms and feelings sound familiar, then you may be an unsuspecting victim of the parasite epidemic that is affecting millions of Americans. It is an epidemic that knows no territorial, economic, or sexual boundaries. It is a silent epidemic of which most doctors in this country are not even aware. Yet according to parasite expert and medical researcher Louis Parrish, M.D., at least eight out of ten of his patients have some kind of parasite infection.

Here is the untold story that finally solves the mystery of many chronic health disorders. It is a story that began for me back in 1974 when I stumbled upon the connection between parasites and disease. In that year, at a special class for the study of "scientific nutrition" in Albuquerque, New Mexico, instructor Hazel Parcells, D.C., N.D., Ph.D., introduced the topic of worms in a most visual manner. She showed the class various preserved specimens of internal visitors that had been passed by patients undergoing treatment for a wide array of unresolved health problems. I have never forgotten the sight of those little bottles and what was in them. For the next two years, I refused to eat in any restaurants—for reasons you will read about later in this book. But most importantly, what I learned from Dr. Parcells was that worms, from the microscopic amoeba to the feet-long tapeworm, are a fundamental root cause of disease and are associated with health problems that go far beyond gastrointestinal tract disturbances.

Since then, in my own nutritional practice, I have observed that many unexplained health conditions often disappeared when parasites were eliminated from the body. These conditions included environmental illness, skin problems, digestive problems, excessive fatigue, hypoglycemia, arthritic-like aches and pains, long-standing obesity, and even depression. Painstaking examination of my clients' food habits, favorite ethnic restaurants, lifestyle, and travel records often revealed the source of infection. I was amazed to find that a patient's travel history was often the missing key to unlocking the underlying cause of persistent flu-like symptoms, allergy, fatigue, gas, and intermittent constipation and diarrhea. Frequently, symptoms started shortly after a vacation to tropical islands, Asia, or South America or a camping trip in Colorado.

A central problem in solving the parasite puzzle is that many parasite-based illnesses can mimic diseases more familiar to the doctor. Roundworm infection, for example, has been misdiagnosed as peptic ulcer and amoebic colitis is often mislabeled as ulcerative colitis. Chronic fatigue syndrome and yeast infection may really be a case of chronic giardiasis, while diabetes and hypoglycemia can be caused by tapeworm infection. The majority of doctors in the United States do not recognize parasites and therefore do not diagnose them. This may be due to the fact that parasitology courses in medical schools are usually offered by a tropical diseases department, giving rise to the notion that parasites are primarily a foreign concern. Furthermore, the inability of technicians to accurately diagnose the problem compounds the issue. The parasite's own reproductive cycle, in which eggs or cysts are passed at irregular intervals, also makes accurate diagnosis tricky.

Today, parasites and the diseases they cause are no longer found just in faraway places like the tropics— places that conjure up images of poverty and poor hygiene. Some parasites, like giardia and pinworms, are, in fact, found predominantly in temperate climates. These organisms as well as others have become more prevalent in America because of a number of modern-day factors discussed throughout this book.

The idea of harboring a living organism inside our bodies is repulsive and unpleasant to dwell upon; but learning all we can about our unwelcome boarders is the only way we can discover enough to evict them and rid ourselves once and for all of their presence. This is one situation in which ignorance is definitely not bliss.

KNOWLEDGE IS THE KEY

In this book I will tell you:

- Which twentieth-century factors have increased the parasite risk in the United States.
- What parasites look like and what symptoms to look for.
- How parasites are transmitted through food, water, animals, sexual practices, and day-care centers.
- How parasitic infections should be diagnosed.

In the following chapters, you will find answers to such questions as:

- What are the most effective natural and medical treatments for parasitic infection?
- How can my family and I prevent infection and reinfection?
- What lifestyle and travel precautions should I take?

The answers to these questions and many more may surprise and even shock you. But this book was written to do just that—awaken you, your family, and your doctor to the fact that parasites are alive and well and thriving in America today. I wrote this book because as a health-care professional I am worried . . . worried that so many individuals are not well, even though they are following a balanced diet and a good exercise program, and are unable to find the reason. I am convinced, after dealing with patients for over eighteen years, that one of the major reasons for the chronic ill health we are seeing today is none other than parasites.

After you read this book, I urge you to share it with as

many people as you can. Pass it on to your neighborhood health clinic, the hospital emergency room, your personal physician, and to veterinarians, day-care centers, outdoor clubs, restaurant owners, and travel agents. Education is the most potent weapon against the parasite epidemic. It is my hope that *Guess What Came to Dinner* will become a wake-up call for every individual living in America today.

1
What You Don't Know *Can* Hurt You

*We have a tremendous parasite problem right here in the
United States—it's just not being identified.*

—Peter Weina, Ph.D., Chief of Pathobiology,
Walter Reed Army Institute of Research, 1991

*I strongly believe that every patient with disorders of
immune function, including multiple allergies (especially food allergy), and patients with unexplained fatigue or with chronic bowel symptoms should be evalu-
ated for the presence of intestinal parasites.*

—Leo Galland, M.D.
Townsend Letter for Doctors, 1988

*Make no mistake about it, worms are the most toxic
agents in the human body. They are one of the primary
underlying causes of disease and are the most basic cause
of a compromised immune system.*

—Hazel Parcells, D.C., N.D., Ph.D., 1974

*P*roverbial voices crying in the wilderness? I think
not. Americans today are host to more than 130
different kinds of parasites, ranging from microscopic organisms to foot-long tapeworms. Practically
every imaginable kind of exotic parasitic disease has been

found on our shores—African sleeping sickness, toxoplasmosis, schistosomiasis, giardiasis, amebiasis, filariasis—unpronounceable to most of us, but potentially deadly nevertheless. Even malaria is making a comeback, with cases of this mosquito-borne tropical disease being reported as close to home as New Jersey, Virginia, Texas, and California.[1]

Parasites are an insidious public health threat in the United States today. Insidious because so very few people are talking about parasites, and even fewer people are listening. Insidious because of the common misconception, among physicians and the general public alike, that parasites occur only in tropical Third World countries, areas traditionally associated with malnutrition and poor hygienic practices. Insidious because physicians do no suspect, and therefore do not recognize, classic symptoms. And insidious because even if physicians are aware of the threat, most use outdated and inadequate testing procedures, which result in underdiagnosis.

Lack of education is to blame. In the United States, physicians are simply not educated in parasitology and are, therefore, inexperienced in recognizing common clinical symptoms. A doctor's introduction to parasitology may come from a chapter here and there in a microbiology course in medical school. If parasitology itself is taught at all, it is as a specialty in the department of tropical medicine at some universities. Courses in these departments are not often elected by medical students who believe they will not be seeing "tropical medicine" problems in their general practices in the United States.

Yet times have changed and parasites are much more widespread than previously believed. An article appearing in the June 27, 1978, *Miami Herald* states that a nationwide survey conducted by the Centers for Disease Control (CDC) in 1976 revealed that one in every six people selected at random had one or more parasites. The survey also pinpointed a parasite known as *Giardia lamblia* as the number one culprit in water-borne disease. Louis Parrish, M.D., a New York City physician who specializes in parasites, wrote in 1991, "Based upon my experience, I estimate in the New York metropolitan area that 25 percent of the population is infected. . . . "[2] Projections for the year 2025 suggest that more than half of the 8.3 billion people on Earth will then be infected with parasitic diseases.[3]

Often regarded as opportunistic invaders, parasites have no respect for class boundaries. The publicized illnesses of celebrities like actor Yul Brynner, who became seriously ill from trichinosis after eating in a well-known New York restaurant, and tennis pro Martina Navratilova, who was affected by cat-transmitted toxoplasmosis, illustrate that we are all susceptible. Contaminated well-water at some of this nation's most prestigious ski resorts has led to outbreaks of giardiasis, which goes to show that parasites can occur even in the seats of the mighty.

HOW DID IT HAPPEN?

A number of seemingly unrelated factors unique to the late twentieth century have contributed to the unrestrained parasite epidemic and added to the increased risk of parasitic infection. Some of these factors include:

- The rise in international travel.
- The contamination of municipal and rural water supplies.
- The increasing use of day-care centers.
- The influx of refugee and immigrant populations from endemic areas.

- The return of armed forces from overseas.
- The continued popularity of household pets.
- The increasing popularity of exotic regional foods.
- The use of antibiotics and immunosuppressive drugs.
- The sexual revolution.
- The spread of AIDS.

Let's examine each of these factors in detail.

International Travel

Today more than ever before, American tourists are traveling to remote areas of the world. An affluent society is a mobile one. In 1990 alone, more than 390 million people worldwide made international trips for pleasure and/or business. Over 15 million of them were Americans, and half of these Americans traveled to Third World countries. More adventurous trips to exotic destinations like the Caribbean Islands and remote areas of Mexico, South America, Asia, Africa, China, and Israel have replaced the old-fashioned grand tour. We know that smallpox, cholera, and the plague have been eradicated, so we're safe.

Not so.

Unfortunately, travel can be fatal. As mentioned earlier, malaria, the most virulent of the parasitic diseases, is on the rise both here and abroad. Malaria is a ruthless killer, responsible for up to 2 million deaths per year in over 100 countries. The rise of this disease is partly due to the fact that mosquitoes have become resistant to DDT and other insecticides. And drug-resistant parasites have been found throughout South America, East Africa, and Southeast Asia. In parts of Thailand, the organism is resistant to every known drug, and the problem now presents a medical crisis.[4] There are many documented clinical cases of travelers, including businessmen and foreign exchange students, who had been infected in other countries but did not manifest symptoms until after their return home. In some of these cases, the disease was properly identified but by that time had progressed beyond the point of medical intervention, and the patients died.[5]

For the majority of us, less threatening conditions such as bouts of diarrhea are expected souvenirs of world travel. We pack our Pepto-Bismol right along with our passports and think nothing of it. Unless we go to St. Petersburg, Russia. Formerly known as Leningrad, this is "Giardia City" to visitors who go home with severe diarrhea, fevers, chills, muscle pain, and intestinal bloating. The cause . . . the city's tap water is infected with *Giardia lamblia*, a microscopic parasite. Visitors to Nepal are routinely stricken with severe cases of giardia, unaffectionately referred to as "Deli-Belly." Giardiasis, however, can do more than ruin your vacation. Symptoms of this illness can persist long after the vacation has ended. And it has been known to set the stage for unexplained conditions such as irritable bowel syndrome and chronic fatigue.[6,7]

Besides returning with photographs of the Great Wall of China, travelers there return with internal hitchhikers in the form of roundworms caused by widespread agricultural use of night soil (human waste). Eggs are not found in stool samples until sixty to seventy-five days after initial infection. By this time, they have gone through their pulmonary phase, creating such symptoms as cough, wheezing, bronchial spasms, and increased mucus. Symptoms of the intestinal phase may mimic those of peptic ulcer but require an entirely different treatment regimen.

The International Travelers Hotline of the Atlanta-based CDC warns those traveling to Africa of the danger of bathing, wading, or swimming in fresh water that may be infested with blood flukes that cause a disease called schistosomiasis. This infection not only produces fever and chills, but it elevates the number of specialized white blood cells known as eosinophils and causes abdominal pain with enlargement of the liver and spleen. Often, these symptoms do not show up until four to eight weeks after exposure, at which time the symptoms may be attributed to more familiar diseases with similar symptoms.

Water Contamination

One of the greatest parasitic hazards is contaminated water, not only abroad but right here in this country. According to David Addiss, M.D., a medical epidemiologist at the CDC, fifteen to twenty years ago giardiasis was seen mainly in international travelers drinking from contaminated water supplies and in campers and backpackers sipping from "pristine mountain streams" that were in reality contaminated by infected forest animals or raw sewage. Giardia, that traveling companion from Nepal and St. Petersburg, is still considered the most common cause of water-borne disease in the United States. Surfacing first in the West, it now appears to have spread to the Northeast, the Southeast, the Rocky Mountains, and the California Sierras.

Steven Rochlitz, Ph.D., in his book *Allergies and Candida*, states, "Giardiasis may be a rampant problem in the U.S. today, since over 50% of our water supply is contaminated with it and, unlike bacteria, it is not killed by chlorination."[8] Hundreds of small water systems throughout the country do not have adequate purification systems. And in urban as well as rural areas, streams and watersheds can become contaminated through infected human sewage.

Day-Care Centers

Rampant parasitic infections exist in day-care centers nationwide. When a child becomes infected in any of the ways discussed in this book, he can easily infect others in day-care centers. The Centers for Disease Control has estimated (estimated because exact figures are not known) that every year, day-care centers are the source of nearly 20,000 cases of giardiasis. A recent CDC survey found that in Fulton County, Georgia, approximately 25 percent of all children in day care were infected with giardia; in New Haven, Connecticut, the rate was twice as high at 50 percent; and in Anaheim, California, the rate of giardia in one day-care center increased from 3 percent to 43 percent from 1981 to 1991.[9]

Since the disease can be spread through direct contact with infected feces, day-care centers provide a ready environment for transmission and have been referred to as "the open sewers of the 20th Century."[10] Because giardia cysts lodge under the fingernails, the infection can be inadvertently spread from one infant to another during diaper-changes. It is also spread by inquisitive toddlers touching dirty diapers and then contaminating toys, drinking faucets, and themselves with their frequent hand-to-mouth contact. According to Dennis Juranek, D.V.M., chief of Epidemiology and of The Parasitic Disease Branch at the CDC, roughly 20 percent of parents become infected themselves while caring for their sick children.

Immigrants

Parasitic infection is more predominant in the tropics and the subtropical areas of the world because of climate and unsanitary conditions. Parasites are much more prevalent in immigrants from areas like the South Pacific, Mexico, South America, Asia, and Haiti. Not counting illegal aliens, over 16 million foreign students, diplomats, travelers, and immigrants entered the United States in 1989. During the 1970s, at the end of the Vietnam War, this country was inundated with a massive influx of immigrants from Southeast Asia. Many of these refugees and immigrants come from parasite-infested areas. While they may not be exhibiting symptoms of the diseases, they may still be carriers, just as infectious as those with full-blown symptoms.

Recent immigrants to this country, who often are unskilled and unable to speak English but willing to work for minimum wages or less, very often seek jobs in kitchens where today there are no obstacles to their employment. I have observed that the majority of restaurant workers no longer wear hair nets or gloves when handling food, and often the same person who serves your food takes your "dirty" money. With this lack of basic sanitation in the restaurants of America, the exposure rate to infectious diseases is mushrooming.

Immigrants also find work as babysitters or housekeepers. An Associated Press article that ran on September 3, 1992, carries the headline "Worldly Worms! Traveling Parasites Leave Latin America to Afflict Big Apple." The article goes on to describe how four orthodox Jews in New York City were mysteriously stricken with seizures. CT scans showed pork tapeworm cysts in the brain, a most startling revelation considering these individuals never ate pork due to their religious dietary laws. A Centers for Disease Control formal investigation discovered the single common denominator in every case history—a housekeeper originally from Central America where pork tapeworm infection is relatively common. The investigators theorized that the housekeepers unknowingly carried the

tapeworm eggs and infected the Jewish families by contaminating their food.

Armed Forces

Soldiers stationed overseas can harbor a variety of parasites. More than the troops come home. Headlines such as
"Disease Is Cited in Veterans' Suit,"[11] and "Gulf War Parasite Halts Troop Blood Drive"[12] graphically bring the awareness of parasitic diseases from foreign shores to America.
From 1963 to 1975, thousands of troops returning from
Southeast Asia were carrying parasite-induced diseases
that affected their intestines, lungs, liver, and central nervous systems.[13] In 1985, five Vietnam War veterans filed a
class-action medical malpractice suit against the Veterans
Administration for failing to properly test, diagnose, and
treat them for parasitic filariasis. Filariasis, a disease endemic to southeast Asia, is caused by worms carried by
infected mosquitoes and can lead to swelling of the lymph
glands and a condition known as elephantiasis. Lawyers
and doctors for the five veterans contend that hundreds to
tens of thousands of Vietnam veterans might be suffering
from this disease. More recently, 540,000 American troops
returning from Desert Storm were told not to donate blood
because of the incidence of the parasitic disease leishmaniasis, spread by desert sand flies. Diarrhea, abdominal pain,
and fever are symptoms of this infectious disease. Unexplained illness with fever may be a sign of a new species of
leishmaniasis found in the Gulf vets.

Pets

Pets are hosts to numerous parasites and are unexpected
spreaders of disease. There are 240 infectious diseases

transmitted by animals to humans. Of these, 65 are transmitted by dogs and 39 by cats. There are 110 million dogs and cats living in America's households, making exposure to some of these diseases significant. One pet-food manufacturer says that 89 percent of all house cats in America sleep with their owners. Dog and cat roundworm, hookworm, and cat-transmitted toxoplasmosis can become severe in pregnant women and children and even life threatening in immunocompromised individuals. Phillip Goscienski, M.D., head of the Infectious Disease Branch of Pediatrics at the Naval Regional Medical Center, finds it remarkable that these diseases are almost always unsuspected and unrecognized.[14]

Exotic Foods

The more cosmopolitan the city, the greater the proliferation of exotic restaurants. Our fascination with regional foods has led to an increased incidence of parasites. Exotic foods that are often prepared raw or undercooked pose a significant parasite risk. Shushi . . . sashimi . . . steak tartare . . . ceviche . . . Dutch herring. The CDC 1976 nationwide survey into parasitic diseases pinpointed a 100 percent increase in tapeworm infections in the preceding ten years. Tapeworm is transmitted in raw or undercooked fish, beef, and pork.

Pacific rockfish (commonly known as red snapper) and Pacific salmon are most frequently infested with anisakid worms, although the worms have also been found in Atlantic waters in other fish such as haddock.[15,16] With the increasing prevalence of microwave cooking, fish is frequently undercooked, allowing the larvae to survive and enter the human system. These worms cause anisakiasis (a condition resembling Crohn's disease), stomach ulcers, and appendicitis. Surgical treatment can be necessary in the later course of this disease because of intestinal perforation or obstruction.

Antibiotics and Immunosuppressive Drugs

As mentioned before, parasites are opportunistic invaders. When the intestinal system is in healthy balance, there is less opportunity for parasitic infestation. Antibiotics, however, kill bacteria indiscriminately, both the good and the bad, upsetting the natural ecology of the gastrointestinal tract and vagina. This often leads to yeast overgrowth and trichomoniasis. *Trichomonas vaginalis* is a microscopic parasite that causes foul-smelling vaginal discharge, burning sensation, and inflammation. In some areas of the United States, this condition is found in 50 percent of all women. It is sexually transmitted and when passed to a male partner can cause non-specific urethritis.

The immune system is our first line of defense against invading bacteria, viruses, and parasites. Patients with compromised immune systems or those undergoing immunosuppressive drug therapies for cancer and organ transplants are at greater risk for toxoplasmosis, an opportunistic infection that attacks the central nervous system, heart, and lungs. While the effects of this infection in healthy individuals can be asymptomatic, in compromised patients it can be life threatening.

The Sexual Revolution

The sexual revolution of the late 1960s and early 1970s made it acceptable to have a variety of sexual partners and practices. The increase in the number of sexual partners also increased the likelihood of sexually transmitted parasites, which include *Trichomonas vaginalis, Entamoeba histolyticia, Giardia lamblia,* pinworms, and pork tapeworms. The increasing acceptance of anal/oral sex among heterosexuals has opened the door to the spread of parasite infections because many of these infections are spread to hands, mouth, and body via fecal contamination.

Spread of AIDS

There seems to be a relationship between parasites and AIDS. Parasites may be a cofactor in the development of AIDS. An article appearing in *The New England Journal of Medicine* draws a connection between the disease and epidemic outbreaks of amebiasis two years prior to the San Francisco AIDS outbreak.[17] University of Virginia School of Medicine researchers point out that amoebas produce a substance that ruptures immune defense cells that have engulfed the HIV virus. Once those cells are ruptured, the virus spreads throughout the system. In addition, as a result of the AIDS epidemic, the incidence of many unusual parasitic diseases, such as *Pneumocystis carinii* pneumonia, cryptosporidiosis, and strongyloidiasis has increased. These diseases can be fatal in the AIDS victim.

OUR GLOBAL VILLAGE

As jet travel has transformed our planet into a global village, so too have parasites developed wings. Our current lifestyle habits of traveling, eating out, camping in the wilderness, placing children in day-care centers, caring for pets, and using antibiotics increase the likelihood of exposure to parasitic disease here in America.

On January 29, 1985, the Public Broadcasting Service aired a "Nova" program entitled "Conquest of the Parasites." In this televised documentary, the diseases that parasites cause were referred to as the "great neglected diseases." They are "great" because they affect hundreds of millions of people, and they are neglected by the public, by physicians, and by the political and funding agencies of the world. Although hookworm disease affects about 900 million people worldwide, the world's agencies spend less that $1 million on hookworm research. That's less than a dime per stricken individual, a particularly disheartening figure when one realizes that 60 thousand of those stricken will die. Given the enormity of the parasitic infection problem, it is clear that funding is poorly allocated.

To prevent *you* from "neglecting" the diseases, this book will help you understand the kinds of internal parasites most commonly found in Americans today, the typical signs and symptoms, means of transmission, diagnostic procedures, and methods of treatment and prevention.

2
The Warning Signs of Parasites

Over half of all Americans will at some point in their lives become hosts to parasites, according to health experts.[1] Since the effects of infection reach far beyond the gastrointestinal tract, it behooves all of us to be on the alert for the wide array of bodily symptoms that signal the presence of parasites. Signs and symptoms may come about during initial exposure, shortly after that exposure, or many months later. What many of us are attributing to old age, stress, or plain old poor health may, in fact, be due to an uninvited guest.

The word "parasite" is from the Greek words *para* (meaning beside) and *sitos* (meaning food). Most medical dictionaries define a parasite as "an animal or plant that lives on or in another organism from which it obtains nutriment." A basic element in the parasite definition is that a parasite is "usually injuring" or "without contributing to survival." The relationship that is formed between the two organisms is defined as "parasitism." My concern in this book is endoparasites, which live inside the body, rather than ectoparasites, which live on the body like mites and ticks. The organism that serves as the home for the parasite is known as the "host." The transmitting agent that carries the infecting pathogen is called a "vector."

The human being becomes a host through one of four pathways. The first is infected food or water (sources of roundworm, amoeba, and giardia); the second is via a vector, such as a mosquito (carrier of dog heartworm, filaria, and malaria), a flea (carrier of dog tapeworm), the common housefly (transmits amebic cysts), and the sand fly (carrier of leishmaniasis); the third is from sexual contact (infected partners can transmit trichomonas, giardia, and amoeba); and the fourth is through the nose and skin (pinworm eggs and *Toxoplasma gondii* can be inhaled from contaminated dust; hookworms, schistosomes, and strongyloides can penetrate exposed skin or bare feet). The airplane can be considered another parasitic pathway or vector in its own right because extensive foreign travel has exposed Americans to a whole gamut of exotic diseases never before encountered in their homeland.

Table 1 (see page 24)—which identifies the parasite, size, site in host, portal of entry, source of infection, most common symptoms, laboratory diagnosis, therapeutic agents, and special remarks—will help you see that practically every part of the human body can be affected by parasites. Most invaders inhabit the gastrointestinal tract (mainly the small intestine, but also the colon), with the circulatory system (blood and lymph) following close behind. During the adolescent or larva stages of their migratory life cycle, many organisms can invade the lungs. And organs like the heart, liver, spleen, eyes, and brain are not immune from the damaging effects.

While many of our unexpected visitors may be invisible, their symptoms can be very apparent. In this situation, the old adage "out of sight, out of mind" definitely does not apply. The warning signs for parasites are also symptoms of other common illnesses. For this reason, parasitic infections are often misdiagnosed and ensuing treatment does not result in the alleviation of symptoms or disease. When symptoms continue even after a course of treatment, parasite screening procedures should be initiated. The following are warning signs for parasites: constipation, diarrhea, gas and bloating, irritable bowel syndrome, joint and muscle aches and pains, anemia, allergy, skin conditions, granulomas, nervousness, sleep disturbances, teeth grinding, chronic fatigue, and immune dysfunction.

CONSTIPATION

Some worms, because of their shape and large size, can physically obstruct certain organs. Heavy worm infections can block the common bile duct and the intestinal tract, making elimination infrequent and difficult.

DIARRHEA

Certain parasites, primarily protozoa, produce a prostaglandin (hormonelike substances found in various human tissues) which creates a sodium and chloride loss that leads to frequent watery stools. The diarrhea process in parasite infection is, therefore, a function of the parasite, not the body's attempt to rid itself of an infectious organism.

GAS AND BLOATING

Some parasites live in the upper small intestine where the inflammation they produce causes both gas and bloating.

Table 1. Protozoan Infections of Man

The information in this table can assist you and your doctor in identifying and treating parasitic diseases. Note that the "site in host" refers to the part of the body in which the parasite "resides" permanently. Parasites normally migrate to this point after entering the host through the "portal of entry." When parasites are present in a human host, they produce a wide variety of symptoms, which can be as general as fever, chills, or intestinal

	Common Name of Parasite or Disease	Length of Parasite	Site in Host	Portal of Entry
NEMATHELMINTHES	**ROUNDWORMS**			
Necator americanus	New World or tropical hookworm Uncinariasis	To 1.1 cm	Small intestine, attached	Skin, usually feet
Ancylostoma duodenale	Old world hookworm Ancylostomiasis	To 1.3 cm		
Ancylostoma braziliense	Creeping eruption, cutaneous larva migrans (hookworm larva)	To 0.3 mm (larva)	Intradermal	Skin
Ascaris lumbricoides	Large roundworm	To 35 cm	Small intestine	Mouth
Toxocara canis *T. cati*	Visceral larva migrans	0.3 mm (larva)	Liver, lung, brain, eye	Mouth
Enterobius vermicularis	Pinworm, seatworm, Oxyuris	To 1.3 cm	Large intestine, appendix	Mouth
Trichuris trichiura	Whipworm, threadworm	To 5.0 cm	Caecum, large intestine, ileum	Mouth
Trichinella spiralis	Trichinosis	To 0.4 cm	Adult: small intestine wall. Encysted larva: striated muscle	Mouth

problems. *Diagnosis cannot, therefore, be based upon symptomatology. Accurate diagnosis and identification of the parasite can be made only if the proper laboratory tests are administered and reliably interpreted. Treatment may then include surgical and/or nutritional measures as well as drugs (see the appendix for specific drug recommendations).*

Source of Infection, Intermediate Host or Vector	Most Common Clinical Symptoms	Laboratory Diagnosis	Therapeutic Agent	Remarks
Infective filariform larvae in soil	Anemia, growth retardation, G.I. symptoms	Eggs in stool	Pyrantel pamoate Bephenium-hydroxynaphthoate Tetrachlorethylene Thiabendazole	Prophylaxis by excreta disposal. Iron therapy important in blood regeneration
Dog and cat hookworm larvae in soil	Serpiginous skin lesions, itch	History and physical examination	Thiabendazole ointment, freezing, x-ray	Infection of bathers, plumbers, "sandbox" babies
Eggs from soil or vegetables	Vague abdominal distress	Eggs in stool	Piperazine Pyrantel pamoate	Worms migrate into bile, pancreatic ducts and peritoneum. Intestinal obstruction
Eggs from soil	Pneumonitis, eosinophilia	Hemagglutination, flocculation tests	Prednisone Diethylcarbamazine Thiabendazole	Eosinophilia, anemia, hyperglobulinemia
Eggs in environment; autoinfection	Anal pruritis	Eggs in perianal region. Scotch tape swab	Pyrantel pamoate Piperazine Pyrvinium pamoate	Entire family frequently infected. Personal hygiene important
Eggs from soil or vegetables	Abdominal discomfort, anemia, bloody stools	Eggs in stool	Mebendazole Hexylresorcinol enema	Worm lives many years. Frequently with hookworm and *Ascaris*
Infected pork, cyst (rarely bear)	Orbital edema, muscle pain, eosinophilia	Skin test, comp. fix., flocculation, biopsy	Prednisone gives symptomatic relief Thiabendazole	Thorough cooking of pork and pork products kills encysted larvae

	Common Name of Parasite or Disease	Length of Parasite	Site in Host	Portal of Entry
Strongyloides stercoralis	Cochin China diarrhea	To 0.2 cm	In wall of small intestine	Skin
Wuchereria bancrofti	Filariasis	To 10 cm	Lymphatics	Skin
Brugia malayi	Filariasis	To 6 cm	Lymphatics	Skin
Acanthocheilonema perstans	Persistent filaria	To 8 cm	Body cavities	Skin
Mansonella ozzardi		To 8 cm	Body cavities	Skin
Loa loa	Eyeworm	To 7 cm	Subcutaneous	Skin
Onchocerca volvulus	Blinding filariasis	To 50 cm	Subcutaneous	Skin
Dracunculus medinensis	Fiery serpent Guinea worm	To 120 cm	Subcutaneous	Mouth
PLATYHELMINTHES	TAPEWORMS			
Taenia saginata	Beef tapeworm	To 12 meters	Small intestine	Mouth
Hymenolepis nana	Dwarf tapeworm	To 4 cm	Adults and cysts in small intestine	Mouth
Hymenolepis diminuta	Rat tapeworm	To 60 cm	Small intestine	Mouth
Diphyllobothrium latum	Fish or broad tapeworm	To 10 meters	Small intestine	Mouth
Taenia solium	Pork tapeworm	To 7 meters	Small intestine	Mouth
T. solium (cysts)	Cysticercosis Verminous epilepsy	To 0.8 cm Brain, to 2.5 cm	Muscles, brain, eye	Mouth
Echinococcus granulosus	Hydatid cyst	To 15 cm	Liver, lungs, brain, bones	Mouth

Source of Infection, Intermediate Host or Vector	Most Common Clinical Symptoms	Laboratory Diagnosis	Therapeutic Agents	Remarks
Larva in soil	Abdominal discomfort, diarrhea	Larvae in stool	Thiabendazole Pyrvinium pamoate	Autoinfection occurs
Mosquitoes	Lymphangitis, fever	Blood smear, night	Diethylcarbamazine, surgery	Elephantiasis of leg, arms, scrotum, breasts
Mosquitoes	Lymphangitis, fever	Blood smear, night	Diethylcarbamazine, surgery	Elephantiasis
Culicoides (fly)	Abdominal pain due to liver invasion(?)	Blood smear	Diethylcarbamazine	
Culicoides (fly)	Asymptomatic(?)	Blood smear	Diethylcarbamazine	
Chrysops (fly)	Local inflammation, transient tumor	Blood smear, day	Diethylcarbamazine Surgical removal	Calabar swelling
Simulium (fly)	Subcutaneous nodules, loss of vision	Skin biopsy, nodule aspirate	Diethylcarbamazine Suramin	Nodules on head and body
Cyclops	Inflammation and ulcers of legs and feet	Lesions, x-ray of calcified worm	Thiabendazole Niridazole	Boil or filter drinking water
Cysts in beef	Usually none	Eggs and segments in stool. Scotch tape swab	Niclosamide Quinacrine Paromomycin	Usually only 1 worm
Eggs from feces	Abdominal discomfort	Eggs in stool	Niclosamide Paromomycin	Numerous worms, infection of children
Cysts from insects	Usually none	Eggs in stool	Niclosamide Paromomycin	Primarily a rat parasite
Plerocercoid in fresh-water fish	Anemia very rare in the U.S.	Eggs in stool	Niclosamide Paromomycin Quinacrine	Prophylaxis by excreta disposal. Cook fish well
Cyst in pork	Usually none	Eggs and segments in stool. Scotch tape swab	Quinacrine Niclosamide Paromomycin	Uncommon in U.S. Frequent in Mexico, Central, South America
Eggs from feces, regurgitation of eggs	Intracranial pressure Epilepsy	Skin test, x-ray of calcified cysts	Surgery	Uncommon in U.S. Autoinfection possible
Eggs from dog feces	Pressure symptoms in various organs	Skin, comp. fix., hemagglutination tests, x-ray	Surgery	Uncommon in untraveled natives of U.S.

	Common Name of Parasite or Disease	Length of Parasite	Site in Host	Portal of Entry
PLATYHELMINTHES	**FLUKES**			
Schistosoma mansoni	Schistosomiasis "Bilharzia"	To 1.4 cm	Veins of large intestine	Skin
Schistosoma haematobium	"	2.0 cm	Veins of urinary bladder	Skin
Schistosoma japonicum	"	2.6 cm	Veins of small intestine	Skin
Fasciolopsis buski	Intestinal fluke	2–7 cm	Small intestine	Mouth
Clonorchis sinensis	Human liver fluke	1–2.5 cm	Bile ducts	Mouth
Paragonimus westermani	Lung fluke	1.0 cm	Lungs	Mouth
PROTOZOA				
Plasmodium vivax	Benign tertian malaria	Intracellular	Liver parenchyma, red blood cells	Skin
Plasmodium falciparum	Malignant tertian malaria			
Plasmodium malariae	Quartan malaria			
Plasmodium ovale				
Leishmania donovani	Visceral leishmaniasis, kala-azar	Intracellular 2 μ	Monocytes, P.M.N., endothelial cells	Skin
Leishmania tropica	Cutaneous leishmaniasis	"	In histiocytes of skin and mucosa	Skin
Leishmania braziliensis	Espundia, mucocutaneous leishmaniasis	"	"	Skin
Trypanosoma gambiense	African sleeping sickness	14–33 μ	Lymph glands, blood stream, brain	Skin
Trypanosoma rhodesiense				

Source of Infection, Intermediate Host or Vector	Most Common Clinical Symptoms	Laboratory Diagnosis	Therapeutic Agents	Remarks
Cercaria in fresh water, from snail	Chronic dysentery, fibrosis of liver	Eggs in stool, rectal or liver biopsy	Stibophen Niridazole Astiban	Africa, South America. Common in Puerto Ricans
"	Urinary disturbances, hematuria	Eggs in urine, cystoscopy	Niridazole Astiban Stibophen	Africa, Middle East
"	Dysentery, hepatic fibrosis	Eggs in stool, liver biopsy	Antimony potassium tartrate Astiban Stibophen	China, Japan, Philippines, Celebes
Water nuts and vegetables	Diarrhea, edema, abdominal pain	Eggs in stool	Hexylresorcinol Tetrachlorethylene Bephenium hydroxynaphthoate	
Fresh-water fish	Indigestion, diarrhea, hepatomegaly	Eggs in stool	Chloroquine Dehydroemetine Emetine	Usually in Orientals
Fresh-water crustaceans (crabs)	Hemoptysis, cough, abdominal pain, fever	Eggs in sputum and stool	Bithionol Chloroquine	Wandering worms in brain and other organs
Anopheles mosquito Transfusions Drug addict syringe	Fever, chill, sweat, enlarged spleen Hemoglobinuria in "black water fever"	Repeated blood smears	Chloroquine Primaquine Sulfamethoxine Pyrimethamine Sulfadiazine Quinine Amodiaquine	Fever irregular in early disease. Incubation long after drug suppression. Drug-resistant strains
Phlebotomus (fly)	Fever, enlarged liver and spleen, leukopenia	Liver biopsy, sternal puncture, comp. fix. test, F.A.T.	Antimony sodium gluconate Pentamidine	Signs and symptoms resemble malaria
Phlebotomus	Chronic ulceration of exposed skin areas	Skin scrapings	Antimony sodium gluconate X-ray, CO_2 snow	Immunity following lesion
Phlebotomus	Ulceration of naso-oral region	Scrape lesions	Antimony sodium gluconate Amphotericin B Cycloquanil pamoate	
Tsetse fly	Fever, rash, headache, spleen and liver enlarged	Blood smear, gland puncture, cerebrospinal fluid for trypanosomes	Pentamidine isethionate Suramin Melarsoprol Tryparsamide	Enlargement of posterior cervical lymph nodes, Winterbottom's sign

	Common Name of Parasite or Disease	Length of Parasite	Site in Host	Portal of Entry
PROTOZOA				
Trypanosoma cruzi	South American trypanosomiasis	Intracellular stages Tryp. 20 μ	Tissues—heart Blood	Skin
Entamoeba histolytica	Intestinal amebiasis	15–60 μ	Lumen and wall of large intestine	Mouth
" "	Amebic hepatitis Amebic liver abscess		Liver	Mouth
Dientamoeba fragilis		5–12 μ	Large intestine	Mouth
Balantidium coli		50–100 μ	Large intestine	Mouth
Giardia lamblia	Flagellate diarrhea	11–18 μ	Upper small intestine	Mouth
Trichomonas vaginalis		10–30 μ	Vagina, prostate	Genitalia
Toxoplasma gondii	Toxoplasmosis	4–6 μ	All organs	Mouth
Pneumocystis carinii	Pneumonia	0.5–1.0 μ	Lungs	Respiratory
Naegleria sp.	Interstitial plasma cell pneumonia		Brain	Nose

Source of Infection, Intermediate, Host or Vector	Most Common Clinical Symptoms	Laboratory Diagnosis	Therapeutic Agents	Remarks
Kissing bug Triatomidae	Fever, spleen and liver enlarged Myocarditis	Blood smear, comp. fix., rat inoculation, F.A.T.	Bayer 2502 Primaquine	Unilateral peri-orbital edema, Megacolon. Megaesophagus
Cysts in food and water, from feces	Mild to severe G.I. distress, dysentery	Cysts in cold stool, trophs in purged stool, serology	Diodoquin Paramomycin Dehydroemetine Chloroquine Emetine Tetracyclines Metronidazole	Consider possibility of hepatic infection
"	Enlarged tender liver, fever, leukocytosis	X-ray, serology, cysts or trophs in stool	Metronidazole Dehydroemetine Chloroquine	Treat intestinal amebic infection
Stool (trophs)	Abdominal discomfort, diarrhea	Stool exam, trophs	Diodoquin Tetracyclines	Often asymptomatic
Stool (cyst)	Diarrhea, dysentery	Cysts and trophs in stool	Tetracyclines Diodoquin	Human and porcine sources
Cysts in food and water, from feces	Mild G.I. distress and diarrhea, weight loss	Cysts and trophs in stool	Metronidazole Quinacrine	More common in children than adults
Trophs in vaginal and prostatic secretion	Frothy vaginal discharge	Trophs in vaginal and prostatic fluid	Metronidazole	Treat both sexual partners
Congenital, Infected meat Oocysts in cat's stool	Chorioretinitis Hydrocephalus Convulsions Mimics infect. mono.	Biopsy, methylene blue dye test, comp. fix.	Pyrimethamine with trisul-fapyrimidines	Cerebral calcification. Asymptomatic infections
Respiratory(?)	Pneumonia	Sputum exam, comp. fix.(?)	Pentamidine isethionate Pyrimethamine	Premature babies. Moribund adults
	C.N.S.		Amphotericin B	Highly toxic

Source: Brown, Harold. *Basic Clinical Parasitology, Fourth Edition.* New York: Appleton-Century-Crofts, 1975, pages 4–11. Reprinted with permission.

This situation can be magnified when hard-to-digest foods such as beans and raw fruits and vegetables are eaten. Persistent abdominal distention is a frequent sign of hidden invaders. These gastrointestinal symptoms can persist intermittently for many months or years if the parasites are not eliminated from the body.

IRRITABLE BOWEL SYNDROME

Parasites can irritate, inflame, and coat the intestinal cell wall, leading to a variety of gastrointestinal symptoms and malabsorption of vital nutrients, particularly fatty substances. This malabsorption leads to bulky stools and steatorrhea (excess fat in feces).

JOINT AND MUSCLE ACHES AND PAINS

Parasites are known to migrate and encyst (become enclosed in a sac) in joint fluids, and worms can encyst in muscles. Once this happens, pain becomes evident and is often assumed to be caused by arthritis. Joint and muscle pains and inflammation are also the result of tissue damage caused by some parasites or the body's ongoing immune response to their presence.

ANEMIA

Some varieties of intestinal worms attach themselves to the mucosal lining of the intestines and then leach nutrients from the human host. If they are present in large enough numbers, they can create enough blood loss to cause a type of iron deficiency or pernicious anemia.

ALLERGY

Parasites can irritate and sometimes perforate the intestinal lining, increasing bowel permeability to large undigested molecules. This can activate the body's immune response to produce increased levels of eosinophils, one type of the body's fighter cells. The eosinophils can inflame body tissue, resulting in an allergic reaction. Like allergy, parasites also trigger an increase in the production of immunoglobulin E (IgE).

SKIN CONDITIONS

Intestinal worms can cause hives, rashes, weeping eczema, and other allergic-type skin reactions. Cutaneous ulcers, swellings and sores, papular lesions, and itchy dermatitis can all result from protozoan invasion.

GRANULOMAS

Granulomas are tumor-like masses that encase destroyed larva or parasitic eggs. They develop most often in the colon or rectal walls but can also be found in the lungs, liver, peritoneum, and uterus.

NERVOUSNESS

Parasitic metabolic wastes and toxic substances can serve as irritants to the central nervous system. Restlessness and anxiety are often the result of systemic parasite infestation.

SLEEP DISTURBANCES

Multiple awakenings during the night, particularly between 2 and 3 A.M., are possibly caused by the body's attempts to eliminate toxic wastes via the liver. According to Chinese medicine, these hours are governed by the liver. Sleep disturbances are also caused by nocturnal exits of certain parasites through the anus, creating intense discomfort and itching.

TEETH GRINDING

Bruxism—abnormal grinding, clenching, and gnashing of the teeth—has been observed in cases of parasitic infection. These symptoms are most noticeable among sleeping children. Bruxism may be a nervous response to the internal foreign irritant. It is interesting to note that in the medical literature, the etiology of bruxism remains controversial.

CHRONIC FATIGUE

Chronic fatigue symptoms include tiredness, flu-like complaints, apathy, depression, impaired concentration, and faulty memory. Parasites cause these physical, mental, and emotional symptoms through malnutrition resulting from malabsorption of proteins, carbohydrates, fats, and especially vitamins A and B-12.

IMMUNE DYSFUNCTION

Parasites depress immune system functioning by decreasing the secretion of immunoglobulin A (IgA). Their presence continuously stimulates the immune system response and over time can exhaust this vital defense system, leaving the body open to bacterial and viral infections.

SUMMING UP

Basically, parasites create damage to the host's body in six ways:

1. They destroy cells in the body faster than cells can be regenerated, thereby creating an imbalance that results in ulceration, perforation, or anemia.

2. They produce toxic substances that are harmful to the body. In cases of chronic infection, the body's immune response can be pushed into overdrive, producing elevated levels of eosinophils. Eosinophils are specialized white cells that normally combat any microscopic pathogen, but when their level is elevated, they themselves can cause tissue damage that results in pain and inflammation.

3. The presence of parasites irritates the tissues of the body, inducing an inflammatory reaction on the part of the host.

4. Some parasites invade the body by penetrating the skin, producing dermatitis. During their developmental stage, other parasites perforate and damage the intestinal lining.

5. The size and/or weight of the parasitic cysts, particularly if they are located in the brain, spinal cord, eye, heart, or bones, produces pressure effects on these organs. Obstruction, particularly of the intestine and pancreatic and bile ducts, can also occur.

6. The presence of parasites depresses immune system functioning while activating the immune response. This can eventually lead to immune system exhaustion.

Not every case of ill health can be blamed on parasites.

But if symptoms persist and reoccur at regular intervals after you've been treated for some other diagnosed ailment, then parasites should be suspected. It is a good idea to keep track of your symptoms and look into the parasite connection with the assistance of an experienced healthcare provider. The next chapters will help you to understand the parasite-based illnesses further.

3
Guide to Parasites

*T*his chapter is a reference guide to the individual parasites. Because it is rather technical, you may not want to read it all the way through. You will find it useful to refer back to while reading later chapters. For the sake of not becoming too technical and academic, I have distilled the most pertinent clinical features of each parasite into a basic general description.

Parasites are biochemically complex creatures in their life history, development, reproductive cycles, nutritional requirements, and disease manifestation. They are categorized according to structure, shape, function, and reproductive ability. These include microscopic organisms (Protozoa); round, pin and hookworms (Nematoda); tapeworms (Cestoda); and flukes (Trematoda). Following is a discussion of each grouping and its outstanding characteristics.

PROTOZOA

Protozoa are invisible to the eye. They are one-celled microscopic organisms, but don't let their size fool you. Certain protozoans, through their intensely rapid reproductive ability, can take over the intestinal tract of their host and from there go on to other organs and tissues. Some feed on red blood cells. Texas physician James Lewis aptly describes one such protozoan as "a microscopic vampire."[1] Some Protozoa produce cysts—closed sacs in which they may be safely transported through food and water from one person to another. In the cyst state, protozoans are safe from destruction by human digestive juices. These one-celled "vampires," unlike their larger relatives, can actually destroy the tissues of their host.

Amoeba

Several varieties of amoeba found in humans are not considered disease-producing in normal individuals. Sometimes, however, virulent strains of otherwise non-pathogenic amoeba like *Entamoeba coli* and *Entamoeba hartmanni* can produce mild diarrhea and dysentery. Along with the *Acanthamoeba*, which can cause corneal ulcers in individuals who use tap water for sterilizing contact lenses, the amoeba listed here are the protozoans most commonly found to cause disease.

Entamoeba histolytica

This Protozoa is transmitted in cyst form from fecally contaminated food or water, via an infected food handler, or by flies and cockroaches. *Entamoeba histolytica* has a two-phase life cycle: the infective cyst and the latter trophozoite, which is motile and active. When cysts are ingested, they are first carried to the small intestine, where they are released as trophozoite to the colon. The trophozoite form of the parasite dwells primarily inside the bowel lumen, where it grows and multiplies. The incubation period varies from a few days up to three months. Changes in the host's resistance or the organism's pathogenicity can lead to tissue invasion. The trophozoite can then penetrate through the intestinal lining and invade the liver, lungs, brain, and heart.

Most cases of amebiasis do not produce clinical symptoms. Subclinical symptoms include right-upper quadrant pain, cramps, and occasional nausea and loose stools. In more serious cases, pronounced abdominal distention, dysentery, fever, and hepatitis may result. Extreme infection can cause abscesses in the liver, lungs, and even the brain. Chronic diarrhea, gas, and massive food and environmental allergies have all been reported when amoebas are found in the system. Amebic hepatitis can be mistaken for viral hepatitis; genital amebiasis for carcinoma; amebic colitis for ulcerative colitis; and amebiasis in the brain for brain tumor.

Endolimax nana

This amoeba cousin is a relatively new member of the bad-guy group of Protozoa, according to some researchers. It is the smallest of the intestinal amoebas, and the most convincing research of its underestimated virulence comes from Roger Wyburn-Mason, M.D., Ph.D., a British researcher who wrote *The Causation of Rheumatoid Disease and Many Human Cancers: A New Concept in Medicine* (see Suggested Reading List). Mason's book suggests that *Endolimax nana* is the cause of rheumatoid arthritis and a whole host of collagen-related diseases. This amoeba also lives in the lower bowel and can travel to other parts of the body. Besides the work of Dr. Wyburn-Mason, there have been relatively few reports of *Endolimax nana's* pathogenicity. Some researchers now believe that Wyburn-Mason may have misidentified the amoeba-like organism; nevertheless, they agree that some kind of organism to which many individuals have become genetically susceptible causes rheumatoid arthritis.

Giardia lamblia

Like amoeba, giardia is transmitted in cyst form. The main routes are food and water contaminated by human or animal feces containing the giardia cysts. The cysts can be carried by household pets—dogs, cats, and parakeets. Tap water, mountain streams, and well water are prime sources of contamination. Giardia infection is frequently spread through day-care centers and anal-oral sexual practices. Individuals appear to be more at risk if they have type A blood, lack hydrochloric acid, or have a history of *Candida albicans*.

After the cyst is swallowed and reaches the intestines, it reverts to the trophozoite stage, in which it multiplies by dividing. It adheres to the upper small intestine by means of a sucking disk and coats the lining of the intestinal mucosa, preventing digestion and assimilation of foods and causing a form of gastroenteritis. Following infection, symptoms develop after a one- to three-week incubation period. Symptoms include diarrhea, bloat, foul-smelling gas, nausea, weight loss, heavy mucus, greasy stools, and abdominal cramping. Chills, low-grade fever, belching, and headache may also be present. After the initial episode, the symptoms may diminish, with intermittent diarrhea and constipation, abdominal distention, and foul-smelling gas persisting. The giardia can sometimes attach itself to the bile ducts of the liver, creating symptoms mimicking gall bladder disease.

Damage to the intestinal villi from the giardia can persist long after the infection is controlled. Problems like chronic iron deficiency, anemia, deficiencies of vitamins A and B-12, low serum calcium, lack of folic acid, fat malabsorption, and lactose intolerance occur with prolonged infection. Chronic fatigue and depression are symptomatic of long-standing giardiasis. In small children and the elderly, severe dehydration caused by diarrhea and vomiting can be fatal. In children, giardia can be misdiagnosed as celiac disease or failure-to-thrive syndrome.

Blastocystis hominis

First classified as a non-pathogenic yeast, blastocystis is now recognized by some researchers as a protozoan. The organism does not have the cyst and trophozoite stages of a typical protozoan, however. Blastocystis infects intestines in the region where the small intestine meets the colon. When the organism is found in great enough numbers in the intestinal tract, its host often complains of nausea, gas, abdominal pain, diarrhea, and malaise. At the Great Smokies Diagnostic Laboratory (see page 101), this parasite is one of the most commonly detected in stool samples.

Trichomonas vaginalis

Trichomonas vaginalis, found only in trophozoite form, is a sexually transmitted organism. However, some infections are probably passed through sauna benches, towels, toilet seats, and therapeutic mud and water baths.

Trichomonas can exist in the urethra, in the endocervical and urethral glands, or in the prostate without causing inflammation. Approximately 25 percent of men and approximately 40 percent of women can be host to the organism without showing symptoms. Foul-smelling cheesy vaginal discharge, painful urination, frequent urination, and small vaginal lesions are symptomatic. This organism is capable of producing inflammatory changes on the bladder, urethra, and mucosal surfaces of the vagina.

Trichomoniasis is commonly recognized as a female problem but should also be considered as a possible cause of problems with the male reproductive tract. Males who suffer from prostate infections or painful urination would do well to consider the possibility of trichomonas infection. Non-specific urinary complaints may have their roots in trichomonas because it is passed between sexual partners.

Toxoplasma gondii

Humans can acquire toxoplasmosis from cats, because the cysts of *Toxoplasma gondii* are passed through their feces. These cysts become infectious within three to four days and remain viable for up to eighteen months. Breathing dust containing infectious eggs is another pathway for transmission. Eating undercooked or improperly cooked meat (such as beef, pork, lamb, and rabbit) is another source of infection. Infection can also be acquired through organ transplants or congenitally.

Toxoplasmosis is a prime example of an asymptomatic disease. It is estimated that up to 50 percent of the adult population in America may be carrying a latent infection.[2] In acute forms of the infection, symptoms resemble mononucleosis and include chills, fever, headache, and fatigue. Chronic-phase symptoms include hepatitis, swollen lymph glands, and, in some cases, blindness. Because of the lymph involvement, toxoplasmosis can be misdiagnosed as Hodgkin's disease. In non-immune pregnant women during the first trimester, toxoplasma can cross the placenta barrier, resulting in blindness, mental retardation, and even death to the unborn child. In immunosuppressed individuals, such as those with AIDS, toxoplasmosis is considered an opportunistic infection and affects the central nervous system, brain, lungs, and heart. Other symptoms of an active infection are encephalitis, paralysis on one side of the body, delusional behavior, and intense headaches that are unresponsive to painkillers.

Cryptosporidium muris

Transmitted via contaminated ground water, farm animals, and the fecal-oral route, *Cryptosporidium muris*, like giardia, is found in day-care centers and is directly related to diaper-changing practices. In healthy patients, the infection is usually mild and of short duration. Symptoms include abdominal discomfort, weight loss, fever, and nausea. Long known to cause diarrhea in animals, these organisms have now been identified as a major cause of diarrhea in humans. In immunocompromised individuals, particularly those with AIDS, *cryptosporidium muris* has a life-threatening potential because it can cause severe dehydration and electrolyte imbalances.

Pneumocystis carinii

Acquired by the respiratory route, spores from this widespread organism are inhaled into the body. The trophozoites attach themselves to pulmonary tissue cells. Symptoms include dry cough, fever, weight loss, fatigue, night sweats, and difficulty breathing. This amoeba creates a kind of pneumonia that often causes death by asphyxiation in immunocompromised patients and premature babies.

Plasmodium malariae, Plasmodium ovale, Plasmodium vivax, Plasmodium falciparum

Four kinds of plasmodium, one-celled Protozoa, infect humans. Because they cause malaria, these Protozoa may be the most widely recognized. There are several types of malaria, all transmitted by the bite of an infected Anopheles mosquito.

Once established, the organism invades the red blood cells and destroys them. Malaria can take from four weeks to several months to develop. This is why it is essential to continue protective medication for at least a month after leaving an endemic area. Initially, patients exhibit high fever, shaking, chills, and other flu-like symptoms. Attacks of chills, high fever, and severe sweating can occur every forty-eight or seventy-two hours. Unexplained, recurring fever, malaise, headache, anemia and enlarged liver and spleen are the most common chronic symptoms. Death can result from multi-system failure, including renal failure and ruptured spleen.

Malaria can be of the acute malignant type or the chronic relapsing type. Malaria is most commonly found in Africa, South America, and Southeast Asia. Recent cases have been reported in New Jersey and Rhode Island, with an annual outbreak reported in San Diego.

Leishmania donovani, Leishmania tropica, Leishmania braziliensis

These parasitic Protozoa enter their hosts through the

skin and grow to approximately 2 microns (roughly
.000078 inches). Leishmaniasis, the parasitic disease
found in the troops returning from Desert Storm, is transmitted by sand flies. There are two types of disease manifestations—one consists of frequently ulcerated skin or
mucosal lesions; the other, more serious one infects the
internal organs, like the lymph nodes, liver, bone marrow, and spleen. This disease is most commonly found in
Africa, Latin America, India, and the Middle East.

NEMATODA

This section will introduce you to the larger parasites,
commonly known as worms. While the Protozoa are only
single-celled, these creatures are multicellular. The adult
worms multiply by producing eggs called ova or larvae.
The eggs usually become infectious in soil or in an intermediate host before humans are infected. It is interesting to note that unless the worm infestation is heavy,
many individuals do not show signs of disease. While it
may be unpleasant to consider, it is true that the human
host can co-exist quite comfortably with a few worms,
unless they reproduce in great numbers and create organ obstruction.

Roundworm (*Ascaris lumbricoides*)

The most common intestinal parasite in the world is the
large roundworm known as the *Ascaris lumbricoides*. About
1 billion people are infected with ascaris. Due to their oral
tendencies, children are very prone to roundworm. The
worm resembles the common earthworm in appearance
and is spread directly to humans from soil or food contaminated with human feces. It is found worldwide and is

more common in tropical and subtropical areas, especially in Asia because of the use there of night soil (human excrement) as fertilizer.

Once the worms develop in the human system, they can pass through the liver and lungs, where they create severe tissue irritation and allergic reactions. Adult worms can travel through the body and end up in the liver, heart, and lungs. They can create intestinal obstruction when present in large enough numbers. Symptoms in children include nervousness, colic, poor appetite, failure to thrive, allergic reactions, coughing, and wheezing. Malnutrition in children is also characteristic of heavy ascaris infection because the worms compete for food. Ascaris inhibits absorption of proteins, fats, and carbohydrates. Adults can exhibit vague abdominal pain, edema (abnormal accumulation of fluid) of the lips, allergic reactions, insomnia, anorexia, and weight loss.

Hookworm (*Necator americanus, Ancylostoma duodenal*)

Hookworm larvae are found in warm moist soil. They enter the body by penetrating the skin and are often found in people who frequently go barefoot. Hookworms travel through the bloodstream to the lungs, into the alveoli, and up the trachea to the throat where they are swallowed and end up in their final habitat, the small intestine, in about seven weeks. When the larvae pass through the lungs, bronchitis may develop. The teeth-like hooks of the larvae attach to the intestinal mucosa and rob the body of large amounts of blood. Found worldwide in warm, moist tropical areas, hookworms in the United States are most prevalent in the southeastern part of the country.

The first symptom of hookworm infection is itchy

patches of skin, pimples and/or blisters known as ground itch (dew itch). Other symptoms include itching at entry site, nausea, dizziness, pneumonitis, anorexia, weight loss, and anemia. These worms can live up to fifteen years in the human body.

Pinworm *(Enterobius vermicularis)*

The most common of all the worms in the United States, the pinworm is most prevalent in children. Transmission occurs through contaminated food, water, and house dust as well as human-to-human contact. The adult female pinworm moves outside the anus to lay eggs. These eggs are often transferred by a child's fingers from the itching anal area to the mouth. Children can easily transmit the worms to the entire family through the bathtub, toilet seat, and bedclothes.

Perianal itching is the most classic pinworm symptom. But these little quarter-inch mobile worms that resemble threads have been connected to an enormous range of neurological and behavioral symptoms. Pediatrician Leo Litter, in a ten-year study of over 2,000 cases of children with pinworms, documented seemingly unrelated symptoms that previously had not been associated with this parasitic infection. Some of the more unusual symptoms include abnormal EEGs (electroencephalograms)—sometimes resembling those in cases of brain tumor—epilepsy, hyperactivity, and vision problems. (Dr. Litter's article is listed on page 159. If you have children, or teach, please read it.)

Strongyloides *(Strongyloides stercoralis)*

This nematode is unique because the mature adult can reproduce entirely in the human host or grow into a free-living worm in soil. Strongyloides produce autoinfection in the host and can remain in the body for more than thirty years. Found in Southeast Asia and the southeastern part of the United States, this parasite is extremely difficult to diagnose. The infection is transmitted when larvae penetrate the human through the skin, pores, or hair follicles. Most commonly, invasion occurs between the toes or at the bottom of the foot. The larvae then reach maturity in the intestines. When the larvae invade tissue (primarily the intestinal wall and lung), a condition known as disseminated strongyloides develops; this condition can be fatal.

Abdominal bloating and gastrointestinal problems (including diarrhea and greasy stools) are the primary symptoms. Infections have been known to last up to thirty-six years with the predominant symptoms being nausea, bloating, diarrhea, and pulmonary disorders. This parasitic condition is often found in AIDS victims.

Trichinella *(Trichinella spiralis)*

Just about any symptom known to man can be caused by the various stages of trichinosis infection, which can masquerade as at least fifty more familiar diseases ranging from flu to generalized and specific aches and pains. Most roundworms are transmitted through soil contaminated by feces, but the small spiral-shaped trichinella found in pork is the exception. These tiny roundworms can become enclosed in a cyst inside the muscles of bear, walrus, or pig. If pork is eaten and not thoroughly cooked, the cysts are dissolved by the host's digestive juices, and the worms mature and travel to the muscles, where they become encased. Eventually, the worms can burrow themselves into the larynx, chest, diaphragm, abdomen, jaws, and upper arms. Then they calcify, causing severe muscle soreness and fever.

The symptoms of trichinosis change according to the progress the trichinella make through the body. During the first week of infection, acute diarrhea, nausea, vomiting, and colic occur as the larvae penetrate the first part of the small intestine. Then, when the larvae migrate to muscle tissue, about two to four weeks after the infected meat was eaten, the most classical symptom, severe muscle pain, is experienced. When the larvae finally encyst themselves in muscle fiber, extreme dehydration and toxic edema can be caused. Edema of the lip, face, or eyelids, difficulty in breathing or speaking, chewing problems, enlarged lymph glands, meningitis, and encephalitis can take place. Brain damage, pneumonia, pleurisy, and nephritis are further complications of this disease.

Anisakine Larvae

Anisakid worms have a two-host life cycle: the adult lives in sea mammals, and the infected larval stages appear in fish like Pacific salmon, Pacific rockfish (red snapper), herring, cod, and haddock. Humans become infected by consuming raw, pickled, or smoked herring, or by eating undercooked fish—a common occurrence when relying on the microwave. Symptoms include appendicitis, Crohn's disease, and intestinal inflammation. Sometimes the worms have to be surgically removed because of perforation.

Dog and Cat Roundworm (*Toxocara canis, Toxocara cati*)

Toxocara canis and *Toxocara cati* are dog and cat roundworms that cause a disease called visceral larva migrans

in humans, mainly children. Food, water, and soil contaminated with roundworm eggs are the most common
routes of infection. Children are the most common victims of this malady because of their hand-to-mouth habits
and because their play areas may be contaminated by
roundworm eggs from dogs and cats.

The human is not a viable host for the mature dog or
cat worm, but the immature form causes visceral larva
migrans. When the larvae hatch, they travel to various
parts of the body like the lungs, liver, brain, or eye. They
cause enlarged liver, abdominal pain, and often pneumonitis. A high eosinophil count as well as anemia are
typical of this problem.

**Filaria (*Wuchereria bancrofti, Brugia malayi,
Onchocerca volvulus, Loa loa, Mansonella streptocerca,
Mansonella perstans, Mansonella ozzardi*)**

Including dog heartworm, there are eight species of
filariae known to infect people. Transmitted by blood-
sucking insects and flies, the filariae are microscopic
roundworms that cause diseases endemic to tropical Africa, Southeast Asia, and the South Pacific. The lymphatic
filariae—*Wuchereria bancrofti* and *Brugia malayi*—invade
the bloodstream and lymphatics with pronounced effects
ranging from simple fever and lymph node infection to
deformities like elephantiasis of the legs, arms, scrotum,
and breasts. *Onchocerca volvulus* causes dermatitis, subcutaneous nodules, and eye lesions. In some areas of West
Africa, almost 30 percent of all adults are blind because of
this parasite. Onchocerciasis is known as "river blindness" because the disease occurs in Africa near rivers
where the vector flies breed. Other filarial infections include *Loa loa*, characterized by temporary loss of vision

and transient swellings. All three species of the *Mansonella* filariae cause a type of itching dermatitis.

Dog Heartworm *(Dirofilaria immitis)*

The most endemic areas in the United States for human dog heartworm infection are the Mississippi River Valley and the Atlantic and Gulf Coasts. Man is not a viable host for the fully mature worm; it is the heartworm larvae that invade man. The parasite, which is transmitted by an infected mosquito, usually remains in subcutaneous tissue. The larvae rarely complete their life cycle, but if they do, they migrate to the lung where they become localized in a coin-like lesion. The symptoms are generally mild, with an occasional cough. The major problem is that on an X-ray the lesion can be mistaken for cancer, leading to unnecessary surgery.

CESTODA

The tapeworms are the largest of the intestinal inhabitants of man. They each have a scolex, or head, that attaches to the intestinal wall. As long as the head remains attached to the intestinal mucosa, a new worm can grow from it. Tapeworms do not contain digestive tracts but get their nourishment by absorbing partially digested substances from the host. They are whitish in color, flat, and ribbon-like, with a covering that is a transparent skin-like layer.

Beef Tapeworm *(Taenia saginata)*

Beef tapeworm can be ingested from raw or undercooked beef (rare or medium rare). Despite its size, several feet

long, the beef tapeworm does not produce marked symptoms. It is composed of 1,000- to 2,000-segment strands.
The segment known as the proglottid, which contains both
male and female reproductive organs, bears the eggs.
Tapeworms thrive on the diet of the host for their carbohydrates but utilize the tissues of the host for proteins.

Beef tapeworms have a life span in the intestine of
twenty to twenty-five years. Usually, only one worm at a
time infects the system. Because the worm's presence produces few symptoms, it is rather surprising when the proglottids move out of the anus unexpectedly as they sometimes do. Symptoms such as diarrhea, abdominal cramping,
nervousness, nausea, and loss of appetite are possible.

Pork Tapeworm *(Taenia solium)*

Pork tapeworm is similar to beef tapeworm but is shorter,
with less than 1,000 proglottids. Pork tapeworm infects
man through the eating of infested, undercooked pork
such as fresh or smoked ham or sausage. Unlike the beef
tapeworm, pork tapeworm infection is usually caused by
multiple worms rather than just one. The larva stage develops in the muscle, spreads through the central nervous
system into other tissues and organs, and finally hooks
onto the upper small intestine.

Pork tapeworm causes great harm to the human host
when the immature larvae invade the muscles, heart,
eyes, or brain. The larval migration of pork tapeworm
represents the most dangerous infection of all the tapeworms. In the brain, the worms can create a condition
known as cysticercosis, which can produce seizures and
brain deterioration and often is misdiagnosed as epilepsy.

Fish Tapeworm *(Diphyllobothrium latum)*

This tapeworm, the largest parasite found in humans with up to 4,000 proglottids, is commonly found in Scandinavia, Russia, Japan, Australia, the Great Lakes, Canada, and Alaska. It can be contracted by eating raw or lightly cooked freshwater or certain migratory species of fish, such as Alaskan salmon, perch, pike, pickerel, and American turbot. In the intestine, fish tapeworm can consume 80 to 100 percent of the host's vitamin B-12. A striking vitamin B-12 deficiency or pernicious anemia is the most debilitating effect. Digestive disturbances—including pain and fullness in the upper abdomen, nausea, and anorexia—are common symptoms.

Dog Tapeworm *(Dipylidium caninum)*

Dog tapeworm is transmitted by infected dog fleas. Of all human hosts, children are the most common. By kissing dogs or by having the dogs "kiss" them, children may accidentally swallow an infected dog flea. Called the "pumpkin seed tapeworm," the first hint of its infection may be finding pumpkin-seed-like particles in the stool of the child or in his or her undergarments. These particles are actually the egg-bearing segments (proglottids) of the tapeworm. After the flea is swallowed, the larva is liberated, and in twenty days, the worm reaches maturity. Symptoms are vague but include restlessness and persistent diarrhea.

TREMATODA

Trematoda are leaf-shaped flatworms also known as flukes. They are parasitic during nearly all of their life cycle forms. The cycle begins when larvae are released into freshwater by infected snails. The free-swimming larvae can then directly penetrate the skin of the human host or are ingested after encycsting in or on various edible vegetation, fish, or crustaceans.

Blood Fluke (*Schistosoma japonicum, Schistosoma mansoni, Schistosoma haematobium*)

There are three primary species of blood flukes, or schistosomes, that cause disease. One of the three types of resulting diseases, *Schistosomiasis mansoni*, occurs in Africa, the Eastern Mediterranean, the Caribbean, and South America. Another, *Schistosomiasis japonicum*, is found in Asia. The third, *Schistosomiasis haematobium*, is found in Egypt. Freshwater snails play intermediate host in the life cycle development of these blood flukes. The snails release larvae into water, where the larvae can directly penetrate the skin of swimmers or bathers in contaminated rivers or streams.

The parasite burrows into the skin and is carried through the bloodstream to the veins of the liver, intestines, or bladder. In two forms of schistosomiasis, inflammation begins when the worms lodge in the lining of the intestine or liver. In another form, the bladder and urinary tract can become fatally infected by worms lodged in the walls of the bladder.

Liver Fluke (*Clonorchis sinensis*)

Common in the Orient and Hawaii, the liver fluke is transmitted through the ingestion of raw, dried, salted, pickled, or undercooked fish. Snails, carp, and forty additional species of fish have been known to be intermediate hosts to this fluke. In the human, it inhabits the bile ducts of the liver, causing the liver to become enlarged and tender. It also causes inflammation, chills, fever, jaundice, and a type of hepatitis.

Oriental Lung Fluke *(Paragonimus westermani)*

Found in the Far East, the lung fluke enters the body via infected crabs and crayfish that have been insufficiently cooked or eaten raw. The adult worms go to the lungs and even the brain, where seizures similar to epilepsy can occur. Symptoms include an occasionally mild cough and a peculiar bloodstained, brown, rusty sputum when a victim wakes. The lung fluke can perforate lung tissue and deplete oxygen supplies to the entire bloodstream. Symptoms often resemble those of pulmonary tuberculosis.

Sheep Liver Fluke *(Fasciola hepatica)*

Cases of this fluke have been reported in Central and South America, parts of Africa, Asia, and Australia. Infection is usually acquired from eating the larva worms encysted on aquatic vegetation such as watercress. Worms migrate to the liver and bile ducts, where they produce right-upper-quadrant abdominal pain, liver abscesses, and fibrosis.

Intestinal Fluke *(Fasciolopsis buski)*

Human infections occur mainly in Southeast Asia. Transmission occurs when individuals bite into the unpeeled outer skin of plants that harbor encycsted larvae. Such plants can include water chestnuts, bamboo shoots, and lotus plant roots. Adult flukes live in the duodenum (the shortest, widest portion of the small intestine) and jejunum (connects the duodenum and the ileum, which opens into the large intestine), where they cause ulceration. Symptoms include diarrhea, nausea, vomiting, abdominal pain, and facial and abdominal edema.

As you have learned, parasites are responsible for an enormous panorama of worldwide human health problems. These organisms are very well trained in gaining access to the human body, where they can reproduce through unique life cycle processes that evade our body's defenses. In the next chapters we will examine the invaders' major portals of entry.

4
The Water and Food Connection

*F*ood and water are the most common sources of parasite-based illness. Since most of us eat three times a day and drink water frequently throughout the day, our exposure to these sources is constant. Tap water has been found to be contaminated with parasitic organisms. Both plant and animal foods carry parasites, and cleaning and cooking methods often don't destroy them before ingestion. Today, because of environmental pollution, we all must pay careful attention to the purity of our water and the cleanliness of our food.

THE WATER CONNECTION

In infested waters, mosquitoes and flies can pick up eggs and cysts and transmit them to humans. Sewage sites are also prime parasite reservoirs. Scuba divers and recreational swimmers need to be concerned about the parasite population in freshwater lakes, ponds, and rivers. Divers can become infected with giardia and *Entamoeba histolytica*. In 1983, the scuba divers of New York City who work for the police and fire department had a 22 percent incidence of protozoan infection, probably from the polluted Hudson and East rivers, where more than 188 million gallons of sewage is dumped on a daily basis.[1]

Water is a main avenue for the spread of giardiasis in this country and abroad. For the past several years, the Centers for Disease Control has reported that the giardia organism is the most prevalent cause of water-borne disease in America. According to the Environmental Protection Agency, outbreaks in treated municipal water are doubling every five years. Giardiasis symptoms include diarrhea, bloating, foul gas, nausea, cramping, and intestinal irritation. Symptoms may last for several weeks or months and can even linger on in periodic episodes for years. The exact number of cases in this country remains unknown, since reporting is not required. Because of the number of ignored or misdiagnosed conditions (giardiasis is diagnosed as irritable bowel syndrome and chronic fatigue), many researchers suspect the true number of giardiasis cases is astronomical.

Estimates are that 90 percent of the documented cases of water-borne giardia are coming from surface water that has become contaminated by wild animal feces, such as feces from beaver, muskrat, bear, possum, and raccoon. A few giardia cases have been connected to contaminated water from shallow wells. Giardia used to be referred to as "Beaver Fever," as it was once thought the beaver was the only animal that harbored the cyst. Breakdowns in municipal water systems, particularly in the more mountainous areas of this country, are a major cause of the rise of giardia in America today. Many of these water supplies are supported by reservoirs that rely on back country streams and lakes.

Giardia

Giardia has been found in the waters of the Cascade, Sierra, Rocky, Pacific Northwest, and Appalachian mountains. It has also been found in back streams feeding the municipal water supply of San Francisco. The most widely reported national outbreaks have occurred in Aspen, Colorado; Pittsfield, Massachusetts; Portland, Oregon; Berlin, New Hampshire; Scranton, Pennsylvania; Camas, Washington; and upper New York State. In Rome, New York, approximately 5,000 people became sick from giardia-infected water, resulting in the most serious recent outbreak of giardia in this country. The September–October 1991 issue of *In Health* reports that Pennsylvania leads the country in cases of water-borne disease. Between 1979 and 1990, 15,508 cases of giardia were reported in Pennsylvania. Who knows how many more cases occurred there but were misdiagnosed and not reported? This same article also reports dramatic increases in giardia in New York State, Wisconsin, Washington State, and Vermont, where giardia is now the leading water-borne disease.[2]

With the increasing development of recreational areas along reservoirs that supply public drinking water, the problem may be growing. People who are infected and use these recreational facilities for boating, fishing, or swimming might further contaminate what comes out of our faucets.

Giardia is a tiny organism. About 8,000 trophozoites can fit on the head of a pin. Without a microscope, a person cannot tell if water is infected. No matter how pristine the water source may seem, isolated and remote streams, rivers, and lakes can become contaminated with animal waste. Therefore, all hikers, campers, bikers, hunters, and swimmers should always refrain from drinking wilderness water unless it is properly treated.

Giardia cysts are very hearty and can exist up to three months in cold or tepid water. They are not always killed by chlorination, the most common chemical treatment used for water purification in municipal water supplies. They can be destroyed by iodine-based compounds. However, if the water temperature is close to freezing or contains a great deal of organic material, the amount of iodine necessary to inactivate the cysts makes the water unpalatable. Two commercially available water purification products that are iodine-based and designed for travelers, backpackers, hikers, and campers are Globaline and Polar Pure. Iodine has additional drawbacks. It can cause accidental poisoning and may be contraindicated in sensitive or allergic individuals.

It seems that boiling and filtration are the only surefire ways to kill giardia. At sea level, the water must be brought to a rolling boil and maintained there for at least ten minutes. At higher elevations, boil an additional five minutes. A rolling boil will also kill other protozoans and bacteria. Possibly the most reliable method of purification is through a mechanical filter. The filter must be fine enough to filter out the giardia cyst. The filter size should be no greater than 3 microns (a micron equals one millionth of a meter) because the giardia cyst is approximately 5 microns in size. (See Chapter Nine for specific filter recommendations.)

It is important to realize that giardiasis can also occur by eating vegetables or fruits that have been washed with contaminated water. Unpeeled or uncooked vegetables and fruit should be avoided in areas where giardia is suspect. This precaution, which is generally given to travelers abroad, needs to be observed here in the United States because of the increasing prevalence of outbreaks of giardia.

Amoeba

Another one-celled organism, the amoeba, is also water-borne. The pathogenic form of this microorganism, *Entamoeba histolytica*, causes dysentery, diarrhea, cramping, and a host of other unpleasant symptoms. Only a few amebic cysts ingested from a glass of water are necessary to cause infection. Amebic cysts resist iodine and chlorine purification when the concentrations of these chemicals are too low.

Probably the most publicized outbreak of water-borne disease in this country occurred in Chicago around the time of the 1933 World's Fair. The infection (a form of amoebic dysentery) was traced to the plumbing in a hotel, where a cross-connection had been made between the water pipes and sewage system in an attempt to repair a broken pipe. With the flushing of every toilet, sewage backed up into the drinking water system. About 1,400 people became infected, and 100 people died.[3]

The Acanthamoeba is another type of amoeba found in tap water. It has been known to cause severe eye infections among contact lens wearers who wash their contact lenses in tap water without further disinfection. This infection, Acanthamoeba keratitis,[4] causes pain and inflammation around the cornea. In severe cases, the infection can progress, producing a corneal ulcer, and in some cases necessitating corneal transplant. While relatively few cases have been reported, Acanthamoeba keratitis may be misdiagnosed for other conditions. To avoid Acanthamoeba, all contact lens wearers should use commercially prepared lens cleansing and disinfecting solutions.

Larger Parasites

Water can also contain the eggs and larvae of larger parasites like ascaris, hookworm, and the blood flukes or schistosomes. Particular care should be taken when traveling abroad, not only with drinking water, but with activities like swimming, bathing, rafting, canoeing, boating, and fishing, where direct skin contact can lead to penetration by the blood fluke. Schistosomiasis is a danger in Asia, Africa, and the Middle East, particularly Egypt. This parasitic infection has been reported in American travelers, for example, who river-rafted in African water.[5]

In this country, some environmentalists see the prevalence of giardia and the incidence of other water-borne parasites as an urgent call to action for other toxic problems endemic to our water supplies. With ever-increasing outbreaks of this infection, communities will be forced to update antiquated water systems that not only breed giardia, but deliver bacteria, viruses, lead, and other contaminants to drinking water. The Environmental Protection Agency has set new standards for municipal drinking water systems that draw their water from surface supplies like reservoirs, lakes, streams, and ponds. Guidelines for the new Surface Water Treatment Rule include reducing levels of giardia, as well as other disease-producing viruses and bacteria, to practically zero.

THE FOOD CONNECTION

When parasites are in food, they are almost always transmitted because of improper cooking practices—either too little cooking or none at all. While it is true that the majority of food-borne infections come from animal sources, like pork, beef, lamb, fish, and seafood, vegetarians are not immune. Many plant foods, such as watercress, bamboo shoots, water chestnuts, and lotus roots, may contain parasites in some form. Leafy vegetables, notably lettuce, parsley, and celery, can become contaminated by fertilizers made from human wastes in some countries. For this reason, imported produce from Mexico and other Latin American countries should be thoroughly washed using the Clorox bath described in Chapter Nine.

Pork

The best-known illness caused by a food-borne parasite is undoubtedly trichinosis from pork. Caused by the *Trichinella spiralis* organism, trichinosis can also result from eating undercooked rabbit, wild boar, exotic meats like fox and polar bear, or jerky made from these meats. Polar bear meat infected with trichinella was finally determined to have been the mysterious cause of death in 1897 of three Arctic explorers; thus ended a sixty-year-old mystery.[6]

Trichinosis in this country usually comes from eating undercooked pork. Trichinosis is first transmitted to pigs when they are fed uncooked garbage or when infested rodents, like mice or rats, invade the hogs' feeding areas. A person becomes a host when, upon eating insufficiently cooked pork, the encysted larvae hatch in the intestines and migrate to encyst in muscles. Trichinosis is characterized by a flu-like illness and severe muscle aches and pains, mimicking at least fifty other illnesses.

While rare or undercooked pork can produce trichinosis, fresh, rare, or undercooked pork, smoked ham, and sausage can also carry pork tapeworm infection. The latter is particularly harmful to the body if the pork tapeworm eggs migrate to the brain, where they will hatch into larvae and create cysticercosis, a condition that produces dementia, epilepsy, and sometimes death. The round cyst-like organisms (cysticerci) in the meat make it taste sweeter. Infected pork, because it tastes better, is actually preferred in Colombia.

Pork cooked in a microwave is particularly infective; because of uneven heating, microwaves don't always kill the trichinella. The United States Department of Agriculture recommends that pork cooked in a microwave reach a temperature of 170°F. This is particularly important for the internal parts of the meat.

Beef

Raw beef is enjoyed in the form of steak tartare or carpaccio in some of the finest restaurants of the world; undercooked beef can produce beef tapeworm, a comparatively asymptomatic infection when compared to the harm created by the pork tapeworm. Rare steak and hamburger are risky as well. Undercooked beef or rare pork and lamb can also harbor toxoplasmosis. This disease is said to afflict the fast-food-eaters most of all because hamburgers are so often undercooked or prepared rare. The incriminating evidence can be hidden by mounds of ketchup, mustard, or mayonnaise.

Fish

The parasites most common to fish include fish tapeworms, anisakine larvae, and flukes. Freshwater varieties (mainly white fish) and a few inshore or migrating species like herring, mackerel, and salmon can be contaminated. In Finland, where raw smoked fish is popular, fish tapeworm is quite common, particularly from smoked salmon, causing a characteristic vitamin B-12 deficiency, resulting in anemia and nervous system disorders. Fresh Alaskan salmon is also commonly infected with fish tapeworm, which may be the reason there have been increased infection outbreaks noted in the western part of the United States. Cherry salmon, eaten by the more affluent in Japan for its delicious taste, has evidenced a similar fish tapeworm in that country. Besides salmon, other fish that carry tapeworm include pike, perch, lake trout, grayling, orange roughy, and turbot.

Anisakine larvae often reside in Pacific salmon, Pacific rockfish (red snapper), herring, and cod. When consumed raw (as in sushi, sashimi, and ceviche dishes), partially cooked, pickled, or smoked, these fish can transmit infection to humans. Salmon steaks as opposed to fillets are more likely to contain worms because they come from the abdominal area where more worms reside. Commercial blast-freezing seems to be the most effective way to kill larvae in fish, particularly in salmon and rockfish.

When anisakine larvae are ingested, they penetrate the walls of the stomach or small intestine, causing severe inflammation and pain. The symptoms can mimic appendicitis, gastric ulcer, or stomach cancer. Surgical removal of the worms is often required but can also necessitate removal of infected sections of the intestine. This type of surgery is common in Japan where raw fish is a dietary staple.

Of late, raw fish dishes—especially sushi and sashimi—have become more popular in the United States. In *The New England Journal of Medicine*, researchers have reported finding a new parasite that is transmitted to humans from fish. The Eustrongylides worm had been thought to be found primarily in fish-eating birds. In the case reported in the journal, a 24-year-old student complaining of severe pain in his abdomen underwent surgery for appendicitis. The surgeons found a normal appendix. They also found a ten-inch pinkish-red worm, which crawled out onto the surgical sheets. The student was a once-a-month sushi and sashimi eater and most recently had eaten sushi at a friend's home. The majority of cases of Eustrongylides worm have been reported from homemade sushi dishes, rather than from restaurant preparation.[7]

Because microwaves do not always cook evenly, fish cooked by this method are often underdone and can harbor live parasites. The *Journal of the American Medical Association* reported a case in 1988 of a woman who noticed some "thin, tan, paper-clip-length" worms squirming around in the uneaten piece of haddock she had cooked in her new microwave. Laboratory examination showed them to be anisakid worms.[8]

While this one woman may have changed her eating and/or cooking habits as a result of her experience, an entire nation revolted when they learned of the infestation of worms in native fish. In 1988, the West German fish market virtually collapsed overnight after a monthly public affairs TV program, "The Monitor," aired an episode graphically showing closeups of worm larvae that had been removed from the bellies and flesh of fresh herring. Researchers said they had also found these live larvae in jars of pickled herring on supermarket shelves. The program director, who had aired the show in hopes the fish industry would improve its monitoring practices, was stunned that this one program could so radically change the eating habits of an entire nation.[9]

Liver and lung flukes are more common in the Orient (China, Japan, Korea) because of the ethnic custom of eating raw or insufficiently cooked fish. Liver fluke comes from undercooked, salted, and dried raw fish. It has been found in carp, which is considered a delicacy among Orientals, as well as forty other species. Oriental lung flukes come from raw or inadequately cooked fish such as crabs and crayfish.

Other flukes, such as the intestinal fluke and sheep

liver fluke, can infect aquatic vegetation. Infections are common in China, Thailand, Vietnam, and India. The larvae of the intestinal fluke become encysted on water chestnut hulls, bamboo shoots, and lotus plant roots. The sheep liver fluke in its encysted larvae form attaches to water weeds and watercress, for example. Because these plants are often cultivated in ponds and streams, they can become infected by feces of neighboring cattle and sheep. Such cases have been reported in Latin America, the Middle East, and Australia.

FOOD PREPARATION HABITS

It is not just the eating of food that causes problems. Food preparation habits need to be examined. Since most food-borne parasites arise from raw or undercooked animal foods, the first rule of thumb is to cook. The use of meat thermometers is recommended so that internal temperatures can be checked frequently. This is especially important in microwave cooking. When preparing a meat or fish dish, cooks should refrain from sampling the dish before it is thoroughly cooked. The frequent custom of sampling ethnic dishes (such as country sausage and gefilte fish) for seasonings during preparation can transmit trichinosis and fish worms into the human.

Cutting boards, especially wooden ones, and knives and forks that come into contact with raw, uncooked flesh food—i.e., meat, fish, or lamb—should be disinfected after each item is prepared. The cutting board and silverware can cross-contaminate other foods such as fruits and vegetables. Dr. Hazel Parcells recommends that all utensils used in the preparation of foods (particularly of raw flesh) be cleansed with scalding water or a Clorox bath (see page 128 for Clorox bath formula for all foods). Dr. Parcells suggests using a few drops of Clorox bleach in the final rinsing water for all kitchen utensils. Clorox bleach neutralizes the toxic effects of sprays, bacteria, viruses, and parasites, according to Parcells' research.

Even organic fruits and vegetables should be Cloroxed. Vegetables known to carry parasites include watercress, lettuce, and radishes, as well as leafy greens. Whether the food is organic or not, I instruct all my clients to give all food the Clorox treatment, to be 100 percent on the safe side.

While most people can understand that food and water are common pathways for disease transmission, the prospect that household pets can pass parasitic disease may come as a surprise to pet owners. The next chapter may very well be the most startling in the whole book.

5
Man's Best Friend

*A*nimals, just like humans, can become infected with parasites. Internally, contaminated water and food can spread the problem to our pets. Externally, animals become infected by parasites on their bodies, especially on their fur, because of exposure to infected animal wastes. Forgetting to wash your hands even one time after handling or cleaning up after your animal can transmit the parasite to you. Pets are a wonderful part of life. They provide comfort, companionship, protection, amusement, and unconditional love for their owners. Researchers suggest that people who own animals generally are healthier than those who do not.[1] Yet pets, like humans, are often victims of serious infections that can unintentionally be passed on to their owners. In fact, there is a whole set of diseases classified as "zoonoses" (animal-transmitted diseases) in parasitology textbooks.

Diane Elliot, M.D., a researcher at the Oregon Health

Science University in Portland, wrote in *The New England Journal of Medicine* that humans can become infected with at least 30 illnesses from their pets.[2] Phillip Goscienski, M.D., head of the Infectious Disease Branch of Pediatrics at the Naval Regional Medical Center, San Diego, reported to the California Medical Association that about 40 animal-transmitted diseases have been reported in this country and that infectious diseases transmitted by animals to man total 240. What he found remarkable was that these diseases are almost always unsuspected and unrecognized. He says, for example, that dogs transmit 65 known diseases; cats, 39; and horses 35. And, while a physician would be likely to inquire about contact with animals with an ill zoo employee or experimental laboratory worker, the connection between a sick child and a new puppy is routinely missed.[3]

In 1977, the television program "60 Minutes" discussed children of the Appalachian Mountains who had been infected with a form of dog and cat roundworm that sometimes causes a disease called visceral larva migrans. It was only after the children had died and autopsies were performed that the cause of their swollen bellies, eye problems, and spleen and liver enlargements was found—dog worms.

Whatever the actual number of animal-transmitted diseases may be, the point is clear: animals are major carriers of disease, and most physicians, let alone the general public, are unaware of this fact. Children, pregnant women, and those individuals with crippled immune systems may be the most adversely affected. In an article appearing in the *New York Post* on May 31, 1991, White House physician Dr. Burton Lee "voiced anger at those who say it is nonsense to talk about transmission of disease between people and their pets, pointing to his own experience as a clinician at Memorial Sloane-Kettering

Cancer Center in New York. 'It is not nonsense,' he said, recalling a case where a family's dog got feline leukemia, two children later died of leukemia, and both parents got forms of cancer." New York pediatrician Dr. Stuart Copperman reports that in families where strep throat infection was persistent, the family pets, in 40 percent of the cases, were the carriers of the strep organism. Although the pets showed no symptoms themselves, when they were treated, the strep infections in the human family members cleared up.[4]

There are something like 110 million pet dogs and cats in this country. About half of all dogs may be infected with at least one or more parasites, including hookworm, roundworm, tapeworm, and heartworm. Considering these numbers, the potential for transmission of parasitic infection from animals to humans is high. All pups, for example, are born with the dog roundworm *Toxocara canis.* These roundworm eggs can be deposited in grass, playgrounds, parks, beaches, and sandboxes where toddlers can play and infect themselves by eating dirt or contaminated objects that may contain parasite eggs. Once swallowed, eggs can hatch larvae. While these larvae never mature to full-grown worms in the human host, they do travel to the liver and lungs, and into the circulatory system where they can be passed to virtually any organ.

Dog and cat hookworm larvae can penetrate human skin, forming lesions on the skin at the point of entrance. This syndrome is known as cutaneous larva migrans. Feet, hands, buttocks, and the genital area are the most frequently involved areas. When the larvae die, in a month or two, the disease dissipates. Although not widespread, this disease is more prevalent in the South, where going barefoot makes contact with the larvae more likely.

In the soil, the eggs can become infectious within two weeks. Soil, grass, and shade help the eggs survive. They usually settle near the top of the soil in a silt layer, which protects them from destruction by sunlight. Toxocara eggs are very hardy and can survive for years, resisting the most perilous weather conditions of rain and snow. There are no chemicals that can kill all the toxocara eggs in soil. While contaminated soil is the primary direct source of infection, children can become infected from the coat of a puppy who has been playing in contaminated soil.

PERIL IN DOG DROPPINGS

Toxocara is a constant public health threat in the United States. Studies show that up to 20 percent of soil samples from parks, playgrounds, and schoolyards are contaminated.[5] Toxocara is one of the most common parasites of dogs and cats. It is a highly infectious parasite when you consider the enormous number of dogs and cats in this country. A single female worm can produce as many as 100,000 eggs per day. The environment can be contaminated with virtually millions of eggs since dogs, for example, can harbor several hundred roundworms. All pups are born with roundworm—the most likely reason, by the way, for diarrhea, distended bellies, and lackluster coats. Both dogs and cats can continually become infected as the larvae are passed through the milk of the mother to the baby animal.

How many of us have brought home a young pup to grow up side by side with the kids? Young puppies from three weeks to three months of age create the greatest environmental hazard because they excrete large numbers of roundworm eggs. Most susceptible are children under the age of five, particularly those youngsters between fifteen and thirty-six months.

In the vast majority of cases, there are no symptoms

and dog roundworm infection in humans is self-limiting. I remember a case in which a two-and-a-half-year-old boy demonstrated symptoms of occasional wheezing, coughing, and bloating. A nutrition and health history revealed that the child had a habit of eating dirt and grass. A thorough exam by the child's pediatrician revealed a somewhat enlarged liver. Within three weeks, and without any specific treatment, except my recommendation that the child be supervised to control his dirt-and-grass-eating habit, the child completely recovered.

The disease caused by dog and cat roundworms is called visceral larva migrans and was first recognized in 1952. The disease is characterized by flu-like symptoms, continual abdominal pain, inability to gain weight, blood changes, cough, rash, and enlargement of the spleen and liver. The larvae can migrate through the lungs, muscles, brain, liver, and into the eye. In the more serious cases, tumors can appear in the eye, producing a condition called ocular larva migrans. This is actually a condition of trapped larvae in the retina of the eye. The symptoms include eye pain, strabismus (inability to focus simultaneously with both eyes), and loss of vision. This syndrome may be misdiagnosed as malignant retinoblastoma, resulting in the unnecessary removal of the eye.

Perhaps the best-known parasitic infection of all is the cat-transmitted disease toxoplasmosis, caused by *Toxoplasma gondii*, a very common protozoan parasite. Cats become infected with toxoplasma by eating mice, birds, or raw meat. Through their feces, they then pass the parasite, which can take up to two or three days to become infectious, to man. The oocysts (living eggs) can live up to four months in soil and up to eighteen months in water. Feces may contain potentially viable cysts for up to a year after their deposit. It is estimated that from 30 to 80 percent of domestic cats have the parasite but show no symptoms.

Toxoplasmosis usually produces few or no symptoms at all in healthy older children and adults. It can, however, clinically mimic other diseases such as mononucleosis and lymphatic disorders. Approximately half a billion humans have antibodies to *Toxoplasma gondii*, indicating they have been infected at one time or another with this parasite. Generally, the disease presents no problems except when it strikes a pregnant woman or an individual, like an AIDS victim or a person suffering from chronic fatigue and immune system dysfunction syndrome (CFIDS), who has a compromised immune system.

When a woman becomes infected for the first time during pregnancy, especially in the first trimester, toxoplasmosis can pose a small but significant risk to the unborn baby. Stillbirths, miscarriage, and birth defects such as blindness, cleft palate, hearing loss, mental retardation, seizures, and cerebral palsy can result from congenital infection. Immunosuppressed individuals, particularly patients with AIDS, can develop fatal encephalitis from a toxoplasma infection. For these reasons, pregnant women and individuals with weakened immune systems should have somebody else empty the cat's litter box on a daily basis and should wear gloves when gardening.

Researchers at the federal Centers for Disease Control documented an outbreak of toxoplasmosis in 1977 at a riding stable in Atlanta. Of the eighty-six people who used the stable, thirty-five became infected. Doctors theorized that the disease was spread when stable dust, containing parasite eggs deposited there in cat excrement, was stirred up by the horses and breathed by the riders. Although all the victims recovered, one pregnant woman miscarried.[6] Toxoplasmosis is highly prevalent with over half the population in America infected but asymptomatic. As much as 90 percent of the population in Paris, France, carries the infection.[7] And although cats have been primarily blamed for the spread of toxoplasmosis, our culinary preferences for poorly cooked hamburgers and undercooked lamb and pork are much more likely the source of infection.

Humans are not the only animals who can pick up toxoplasmosis. Dogs can also become infected. They acquire the disease when they eat infected cat feces. Dogs, in fact, often become blind and neurologically impaired by this disease. Thus, it is important to make sure your dogs are not allowed to roam randomly. Keep as watchful an eye as you can on what goes into their mouths.

Other animal-transmitted diseases are connected to fleas. The fleas of both dogs and cats can spread tapeworm if unknowingly ingested by a human. A child's fondness for kissing a pet on the mouth or being licked by the pet creates a risk of swallowing egg-carrying fleas from the pet's mouth. Swallowing infected fleas leads to intestinal infection. Rice-shaped particles that resemble pumpkin seeds in the human's stool may be a sign of dog tapeworm, which can easily be mistaken for pinworms. It is important to deflea household pets frequently.

Dog heartworm can be transmitted to humans by mosquitos. While fatal at times to dogs, dog heartworm is usually benign in humans. Heartworm is most often asymptomatic, although coughing may be a symptom. After humans are bitten by infected mosquitoes, the worm usually remains in subcutaneous tissue. Rarely do the larvae complete their life cycle. If they do, they migrate to the lungs and produce a benign coin-like lesion. On an X-ray, this lesion may be misdiagnosed as lung cancer, leading to needless surgery.

Today both dogs and cats, like most other wild and domestic animals, can also carry giardia. Puppies are especially prone to infection through contact with contaminated water or infected animal waste. Unintentional contact with dog feces can spread the disease to humans throughout the household. Household pets and farm animals can also carry cryptosporidium, a diarrhea-causing protozoa, and contaminate humans.

KEEPING ANIMALS HEALTHY

Taking on the responsibility of a pet is much like bringing up a child. These animals are dependent on you for their well-being. You have to make sure they eat properly; you have to clean up after them and transport them to the vet. In fact, you have to decide if they are sick because, unlike a child, they cannot tell you. Keep an eye out for the classic signs of infection: dull coat, pot belly, poor growth, diarrhea, constipation, vomiting, fatigue, and anemia. Since many parasitic infections in animals, like toxoplasmosis in cats, do not produce recognizable symptoms at all, regular veterinary care is essential to maintain your pet's health.

Keeping your pets free of parasites and fleas is your best protection against animal-transmitted diseases. Prevention is vital in the control of roundworm infection because no chemical can yet kill all the toxocara eggs in the soil. Like humans, healthy, well-fed animals can build up an immunity to many internal parasites. Being well-fed also makes animals such as cats less likely to hunt and eat the animals that carry the *Toxoplasma gondii* organism, like mice and birds. Avoid feeding animals raw meat or raw fish, which harbor tapeworm.

Keep your pets vaccinated and have them periodically screened for parasites and fleas. Routine worming of pets is recommended. Worm at three months, then at six months, and then every six months thereafter. All worming medications contain dangerous compounds. Some pet owners have inadvertently killed their animals by worming them with over-the-counter medications. Don't be taken in by the advertisements for once-a-month over-the-counter products. To evaluate and treat a parasitic condition in your pet properly, a licensed veterinarian is your best bet. The products recommended by the vet will vary depending upon the internal parasite diagnosed and the age and condition of the animal. Repeated treatment is often necessary because of the life cycle of the parasites. The initial deworming treatment is only effective against the mature adults and is not effective against the larvae or immature stages that are still in the animal's body at the time.

Simple common-sense measures can be taken to help prevent the risk of infection for you and your family. Be a "pooper scooper"; don't allow your animals to use the neighborhood as their bathroom; empty your cat's litter box daily; keep it and your animal's food and water dishes disinfected on a regular basis; buy flea collars or use topical insecticides.

Some individuals use pet manure in composting, not realizing the risks involved. Although I applaud the composting effort in general, there are hazards in using dog and cat feces in compost heaps. Composting cannot be relied on to remove the dangers from roundworm eggs. These eggs are very hardy and can contaminate dirt for years. Even after the fecal matter itself is no longer evident, the eggs will still be present. More complete information on preventive measures can be found in Chapter Nine.

It is possible to greatly reduce your risk of infection. If, however, preventive measures fail, you will need the information found in Chapter Six.

6
Are Parasites Your Problem?

U ltimately, each of us is responsible for our own health, and nowhere is this seen more dramatically than in the case of parasites. Parasitic infection remains a neglected disease. Physicians hardly ever suspect parasites as a current American health problem and, therefore, rarely ask for a comprehensive travel and lifestyle history. Without this kind of history, parasites can be easily missed because their symptoms mimic a host of diseases. As mentioned in Chapter One, irritable bowel syndrome and chronic fatigue may be cases of giardia. Persistent allergy is often a case of roundworm infection, while pinworms may be at the bottom of your child's hyperactivity. So a comprehensive personal history emphasizing travel and lifestyle habits is a vital link in determining the primary underlying cause of illness.

The questionnaire in this chapter is a lifestyle checklist designed to highlight the major avenues by which parasites are transmitted into the human body and to identify symptoms that commonly occur in parasite-based illness. This questionnaire can help you, along with your doctor, to assess your parasite risk. This basic questionnaire was first developed while I was working at an environmental detoxification center in San Diego, where parasitic screening was a standard part of total medical testing. Since so many patients were showing positive stool samples and couldn't understand why, the questionnaire helped them trace their sources of infection and pinpoint exactly how, when, and where they may have acquired parasites. Connecting the dates of symptom onset to a trip overseas or a new family pet can provide substantial clues for further health investigation.

Naturally, the more items you check off in this questionnaire, the greater the chances are that your health problems are parasite-connected. But remember, it may take only *one* exposure to tainted food, water, or the bite of an infected mosquito for infection to take place if your resistance is low.

Please answer the questions thoughtfully: "The life you save may be your own."

TRAVEL

☐ Have you ever been to Mexico, Africa, Israel, China, Russia, Asia, Europe, or to Central or South America?

☐ Have you traveled to Hawaii, the Caribbean, the Bahamas, or other tropical islands?

☐ Do you frequently swim in freshwater lakes, streams, or ponds while abroad?

☐ Did you serve overseas while in the military?

□ Were you a prisoner of war in World War II, Korea, or Vietnam?

□ Have you had intestinal problems, unexplained fever, night sweats, or an elevated white blood count during or since traveling abroad?

WATER

□ Is your water supply from a mountainous area?

□ Do you drink untested well water?

□ Have you ever drunk water from lakes, streams, or rivers on hiking or camping trips without first boiling or filtering it?

□ Do you use plain tap water to clean your contact lenses?

□ Do you use regular tap water that is unfiltered for colonics or enemas?

□ Can you trace the onset of symptoms (intermittent constipation and diarrhea, night sweats, muscle aches and pains, unexplained eye ulcers) to any of the above?

FOOD

□ Do you regularly eat unpeeled raw fruits and raw vegetables in salads?

□ Do you frequently eat at sushi bars or salad bars; in delicatessens; vegetarian, Mexican, fish, Indian, Armenian, Greek, Pakistani, Ethiopian, Filipino, Korean, Japanese, Chinese, or Thai restaurants; fast-food restaurants; or steak houses?

☐ Do you use a microwave oven for cooking (as opposed to reheating) pork, fish, or beef?

☐ Do you prefer fish or meat that is undercooked, i.e., rare or medium rare?

☐ Do you frequently eat hot dogs made from pork?

☐ Do you eat smoked or pickled foods, i.e., sausage, lox, herring?

☐ Do you enjoy raw fish dishes like sushi and sashimi, Latin American ceviche, or Dutch green herring?

☐ Do you enjoy raw meat dishes like Italian carpaccio, steak tartare, or Middle Eastern kibbe?

☐ At home, do you use the same cutting board for chicken, fish, and meat as you do for vegetables?

☐ Do you prepare sushi or sashimi dishes at home?

☐ Do you prepare gefilte fish at home?

☐ Can you trace the onset of symptoms (weight loss, anemia, bloating, distended belly) to any of the above?

PETS

☐ Have you gotten a puppy recently?

☐ Have you lived with, or do you currently live with, or frequently handle pets?

☐ Do you forget to wash your hands after petting or cleaning up after your animals, and before eating?

☐ Does your pet sleep with you in your bed?

☐ Do your pets eat out of your plates?

☐ Do you clean your cat's litter box?

□ Do you keep your pets in your yard where children play?

□ Can you trace the onset of your symptoms (abdominal pain, high white blood count, distended belly in children, unexplained fever) to any of the above?

WORK PLACE

□ Do you work in a hospital?

□ Do you work in a pet shop, zoo, experimental laboratory, or veterinary clinic?

□ Do you work with or around animals?

□ Do you work in a day-care center?

□ Do you garden or work in a yard to which cats and dogs have access?

□ Do you work in sanitation?

□ Can you trace the onset of symptoms (gastrointestinal disorders) to any of the above?

SEXUAL PRACTICES

□ Do you engage in oral sex?

□ Do you practice anal intercourse without the use of a condom?

□ Have you had sexual relations with a foreign-born individual?

□ Can you trace the onset of symptoms (persistent reproductive organ problems) to any of the above?

MAJOR SYMPTOMS

Please note that although some or all of these major symptoms can occur in any adult, child, or infant with parasite-based illness, these symptoms might instead be occurring as a result of one of many other illnesses.

Adults

☐ Do you have a bluish cast around your lips?

☐ Is your abdomen distended no matter what you eat?

☐ Are there dark circles around or under the eyes?

☐ Do you have a history of allergy?

☐ Do you suffer from intermittent diarrhea and constipation, intermittent loose and hard stools, or chronic constipation?

☐ Do you have persistent acne, anorexia, anemia, open ileocecal valve, skin eruptions, PMS, bad breath, itching, pale skin, chronic fatigue, food intolerances, sinus congestion, difficulty in breathing, edema, bloody stools, ringing of the ears, anal itching, puffy eyes, palpitations, vague abdominal discomfort, or vertigo?

☐ Do you grind your teeth?

☐ Are you experiencing weight loss or weight gain, loss of appetite, insomnia, depression, moodiness, sugar craving, lethargy, or disorientation?

Children

☐ Does your child have dark circles under his eyes?

☐ Is your child hyperactive?

☐ Has your child been diagnosed with "failure to thrive"?

☐ Does your child grind or clench his teeth at night?

☐ Does your child constantly pick his nose or scratch his behind?

☐ Does your child have a habit of eating dirt?

☐ Does your child wet the bed?

☐ Is your child often restless at night?

☐ Does your child cry often or for no reason?

☐ Does your child tear his hair out?

☐ Does your child have a limp that orthopaedic treatment has not helped?

☐ Does your child have a brassy staccato-type cough?

☐ Does your child have convulsions or an abnormal electroencephalogram (EEG)?

☐ Does your child have recurring headaches?

☐ Is your child unusually sensitive to light and prone to eyelid twitching, blinking frequently, or squinting?

☐ Does your child have unusual tendencies to bleed in the gums, the rectum, or the nose?

Infants

☐ Does your baby have severe intermittent colic?

☐ Does your baby persistently bang his head against the crib?

☐ Is your baby a chronic crier?

☐ Does your baby show a blotchy rash around the perianal area?

If you answered "yes" to more than forty items, you are at high risk for parasitic infection. If you answered "yes" to thirty items, your risk for parasitic infection is moderate. If you answered "yes" to twenty items, you are at risk. If you are not exhibiting any overt symptoms now, remember that many parasitic infections can be dormant and then spring to life when you least expect them. Be aware that symptoms that come and go may still point to an underlying parasitic infection because of reproductive cycles. The various developmental stages of parasites often produce a variety of metabolic toxins and mechanical irritations in several areas of the body—for example, pinworms can stimulate asthmatic attacks because of their movement into the upper respiratory tract.

TYPICAL CASE HISTORIES

While counseling the patients at the San Diego environmental detoxification center, I found that it was only after completing the questionnaire that most patients were able to trace the onset of symptoms to a trip to Mexico or overseas. Oftentimes, the patient was asymptomatic during the trip, then after being home for two to six weeks developed symptoms like massive bloating, gas, and intermittent diarrhea. Because of the delay in symptom development, the trip and symptoms had no connection in the patient's mind.

Had the patients been aware of travel-related parasite risks, they might have taken better precautions in the first place; or if symptoms did develop upon their return, they would have sought immediate medical attention, suspecting the most likely source of their problem. Because symptoms of parasitic infection are so similar to more familiar

and recognizable diseases, making this connection reduces the chance of misdiagnosis.

With the inclusion of a purged stool sample from all
incoming patients to screen for parasites, I discovered
many were being treated for diseases they did not have.
One gentleman, for instance, stated he was being treated
for the past couple of years for peptic ulcer. After completing the questionnaire, he realized his ulcer symptoms began shortly after a trip to China (where human
feces are commonly used for fertilizer). A stool sample
revealed this man had in his system a parasite called
Ascaris lumbricoides, commonly known as roundworm,
which often mimics peptic ulcer. The proper worm medication was prescribed, and the "peptic ulcer" soon disappeared. There are many other problems roundworms
can cause in the body that every individual should learn
to recognize, such as bronchial symptoms, abdominal
pains, and intestinal blockages that can result in chronic
constipation.

Another interesting case concerned a male patient whose
allergy problems became very severe after a trip to Mexico.
Stool testing revealed this patient was infested with giardia,
and soon after medication was given, his allergy problems
decreased. Before treatment, this thirty-five-year-old gentleman was allergic to almost thirty foods and had to curtail his
exercise program and his work because of depression and
severe fatigue. Within several days of taking the prescribed
medication, he was eating foods he had not eaten in years
and feeling like his old self again.

The patient was fine for three weeks, and then the
phone calls to the clinic began again. Our client was beginning to suffer from his old problems. Another stool sample
revealed the presence of giardia cysts. Apparently the
medication had not been strong enough to prevent the
reproductive cycle, and the giardia had taken over his

intestines once again. After another course of medicine, the client was fine, and I believe he is still in good health.

UNUSUAL CASE HISTORIES

Some of the more unusual parasite-related cases I have heard of were shared with me by Dr. Abram Ber, a Phoenix, Arizona, homeopath. A small sampling of hundreds of his cases shows the enormous range of health problems that can be parasite-related.

Case number one concerns a two-and-a-half-year-old girl with a recurring fever of unknown origin and several months' duration. The child exhibited an elevated white blood count and a high SED rate, which shows tissue destruction. She had been taken to several pediatricians, and none could determine the cause of her symptoms. Finally, the mother came to see Dr. Ber. The child was still experiencing a 101°F to 102°F fever, was pale, and showed a poor appetite. When Dr. Ber took a comprehensive case history, he discovered that the child had a number of pets—seven cats and assorted chickens and rabbits—and habitually played naked with these animals. A rectal exam and lab tests revealed pinworms and toxoplasmosis. The child was treated with medication, homeopathy, and immune-boosting injections. Within forty-eight hours, her color and appetite improved, but the fever still persisted. Finally, after continued treatment under Dr. Ber's guidance, the fever subsided and the child recovered.

Case number two concerns a nine-year-old boy with severe behavioral problems and hyperactivity who was brought in to see Dr. Ber. After a complete examination that included testing for parasites, schistosomiasis was found both in the stool and the urine. Puzzled, Dr. Ber asked whether the child had been to Egypt (where schistosomiasis is the number one health problem) or whether the child ate a lot of snails (freshwater snails are the parasite's intermediate host). The mother explained that the child played with snails from his backyard and was not in the habit of washing his hands before eating, despite her pleas. After the proper treatment was administered, the child's hyperactivity diminished and his behavior became normal.

Case number three concerns a woman in her late fifties suffering from such severe muscle pain that she was almost an invalid. Her medical history revealed that sixteen years prior she had lived with a family who ate a great deal of pork. During that time, she developed a flu-like illness accompanied by a high fever. Eventually, this illness went away, but severe aches and pains in the muscles remained. A blood smear showed trichinella, the pork worm that causes trichinosis, while the stool showed *Taenia solium*, or pork tapeworm. After she was treated for parasites, the woman became nearly pain-free.

As these case histories demonstrate, the importance of an in-depth personal history that examines both present and past travel, lifestyle, and dietary patterns cannot be overemphasized. Many diagnostic clues can be uncovered when the health-care practitioner asks the right questions and considers previous travel history in particular. The next chapter explains the newest and most advanced testing methods. Coupling those methods with the information derived from this questionnaire, a health-care practitioner can make a proper diagnosis.

7
Diagnosis

*T*he first step in diagnosing parasites is your physician's suspicion or your concern that parasites may be the root cause of your health problems. This requires a basic understanding of the geographic distribution, methods of transmission, symptomology, and life cycle of parasites. Clinical manifestations related to parasites include eosinophilia (an increase in the number of a certain kind of white blood cell), dysentery, diarrhea, itching, enlarged organs, anemia, and muscular aches and pains. A comprehensive travel, dietary, and lifestyle history is an essential diagnostic tool. The parasite questionnaire provided in Chapter Six can help you or your physician assess your parasite risk.

As far back as 1963, an article appeared in *Medical Tribune* entitled "Parasitic Disease Increases in U.S. from World Travelers Are Reported." In the article, Dr. Martin E. Gordon, a Yale investigator, demonstrates the impor-

tance of a physician's alertness to the geographic distribution and clinical manifestations of the common hookworm
parasite. This awareness can aid in the early diagnosis of
diseases of the modern traveler. Dr. Gordon gives the
example of a Yale freshman with "vague abdominal cramps,
occasional waves of nausea, and a striking picture of ma-
ternal dependence. . . . Knowledge of his eagle scout expe-
dition to Africa the previous summer, when he lived with a
pygmy tribe and walked barefooted, led to diagnostic stool
examination. Hookworm therapy with dithiazanine rapidly
cured his alleged psychoneurosis." Dr. Gordon suggests that
the challenge is to promptly recognize the geographic prevalence of particular parasites and their symptoms so appropriate treatment can be initiated and complications avoided.

A strikingly dramatic example of the importance of
physician alertness is the case of malaria. Reports of malaria here in the United States are on the rise, and strains
are showing increasing resistance to the traditional drugs
used for treatment. "In the United States, many of the
deaths from malaria are the result of delayed diagnosis
and treatment because the health care provider did not
suspect malaria."[1] A thorough travel assessment should
be done on any individual who has a fever and has within
the last two years visited an area where the disease is
endemic. Although most exposed individuals develop
symptoms within six weeks, some may not manifest
symptoms until a year after exposure, and relapses of
malaria can occur up to two years after exposure.[2]

The traditional method for diagnosis of parasitic infection—the search for cysts, trophozoites, ova, eggs, or
worm segments in a random stool sample—is inaccurate
and misleading for several reasons. Parasites that reside
in the tissue and blood, such as those causing malaria,
filariasis, and trichinosis, will not be found in fecal samples. Parasites that are more prevalent in children, like pin-

worms and dogworms (visceral larva migrans), are also rarely seen in the stool. Pinworm eggs are generally not seen in the stool; and since dogworms are in the larvae stage in a visceral larva migrans infection, there are no adults present to lay eggs that could be detected in the stool. To confound the situation further, many parasites do not appear in the stool, because they dwell in the gastrointestinal tract lining (the lumen). These parasites strongly adhere to the intestinal mucosa. Unless they are somehow pulled out from the lining, they do not appear in stool samples.

In the case of some species—*Entamoeba histolytica*, giardia, and strongyloides, for example—cyst, egg, or segment excretion rate can vary from day to day. This is why most parasitologists suggest examination of three stool samples taken on different days. Parasite expert Dr. Louis Parrish even recommends that if these three samples are negative and clinical symptoms persist, three to six more samples should be taken.[3]

However, even when this practice is followed, the diagnosis can be missed. *Medical Microbiology* states:

> Unfortunately, a number of substances that may be administered to the patient in the course of diagnosis or therapy can impair the ability to make a direct diagnosis. These compounds can suppress the shedding of amebas into the stool but may not interfere with the course of invasive infection.
>
> Such compounds include barium, bismuth, kaolin, soapsuds enemas, and antimicrobials that reach the intestinal lumen. The suppression of shedding may be short-lived (soapsuds enema), or may last weeks or months (broad-spectrum antibiotics). *These compounds render direct diagnosis unreliable and often impossible.*[4]

In light of the above, sound diagnostic procedure dictates that a variety of methods be used to determine the specific parasite or parasites present in the body.

CLINICAL TESTS FOR PARASITES

There are many ways to test for parasites. This next section describes the most accurate tests available in laboratories today.

Purged Stool Test

A purged stool test (used with a chemically induced stool as opposed to a random bowel movement) is probably the best all-around general method for identifying the majority of common parasites. This method of analysis is widely considered superior to normal random stool specimens, according to LuCrece Dowell, M. Sc.D., of Dowell Laboratories in Mesa, Arizona. Dowell perfected the method when she was a laboratory officer during World War II. She writes:

> If a patient had a feces examination during the initial or acute phase of dysentery (often amebic) the parasite was usually found and identified. The chronically ill patient with amebic hepatitis or amebic colitis was rarely diagnosable from a random stool examination. These cases were often suspected clinically but repeated random stool examinations failed to confirm the clinical opinion and the patient was considered to have a simple spastic colitis, cause undetermined, or was unjustly judged a malingerer.
> With the preceding problem in mind, a procedure utilizing extensive purging and exten-

sive careful examination was worked out at an Army hospital, based on the invasive properties of one of the more pathogenic parasites, i.e., *Entameba histolytica*. Any type of colitis can be shown due to a pathogen when the stool examination is done on a specimen obtained by proper purging and examination allowing sufficient time.[5]

A purged stool test is particularly good for identifying the presence of giardia, amoeba, roundworm, threadworm, tapeworm, hookworm, cryptosporidium, liver flukes, blood flukes, strongyloides, and blastocystis. The procedure consists of taking 1.5 ounces of Fleet Phospho-Soda on an empty stomach to induce bowel movements. No red meat or red juice should be consumed for at least twenty-four hours prior to the purge. A light evening meal is suggested prior to the purge, and only clear tea or water should be drunk between that meal and the collection of the sample. Dowell found that parasites, regardless of their type, rarely appear before the fourth evacuation, and often as many as twelve bowel movements are required to yield a positive stool or to rule out parasite involvement. Generally, the labs testing purged stool samples will give instructions on which bowel movement to collect for the sample. After collection, the sample is placed in a container with a formaldehyde-based preservative for examination.

A purged stool is contraindicated in cases of gastrointestinal obstruction, pregnancy, appendicitis and debilitation. Since the saline laxative used for the purge is a high-sodium substance, individuals with high blood pressure must be careful. In this case, two to three tablespoons of Epsom salts in a large glass of warm water can be substituted for the Fleet Phospho-Soda.

Bueno-Parish Test

The Bueno-Parrish method, originated by internationally renowned parasitologist Hermann R. Bueno, is a rectal mucus swab combined with specially developed immunofluorescent stains that identify giardia and cryptosporidium. This method is a good alternative for patients who prefer not to use a purged stool or have health problems that would be exacerbated by that method. Rectal mucus is obtained from the mucosa using a small rectal speculum. This simple procedure is easy to perform and has yielded a high positive rate even when the purged stool sample was negative.

A recent study shows that when this method of diagnosis was used, almost 50 percent of patients tested and previously diagnosed as having irritable bowel syndrome were, in reality, suffering from giardiasis. The patients tested had suffered with misdiagnosed bowel problems for an average of seven years.[6]

String Test

If the purged stool and rectal mucus swab prove negative and giardia is still strongly suspected, other tests can be performed. These are the string test (Enterotest), duodenal aspiration, and duodenojejunal biopsy.

The most simple procedure, the string test, recovers a sample of duodenal fluid through the swallowing of a special gelatin capsule containing a string. One end of the string is secured to the patient's cheek while the other is attached to the capsule. After three to four hours, the string is withdrawn through the mouth and mucus is examined microscopically. This method can also be used to diagnose strongyloides.

Blood Tests

Blood tests can be used to reveal an elevated eosinophil count, a general indicator for an infection by parasites— except for giardia and amoeba, which rarely cause eosinophilia. Roundworm, hookworm, toxocara, pinworms, and strongyloides often manifest a high eosinophil count. In fact, roundworm and hookworm can cause up to a 25 percent eosinophilia increase whereas strongyloides may be the reason behind a greater-than-25-percent eosinophilia increase.[7] Many physicians dismiss elevated eosinophils as an indicator of allergy, not realizing the primary allergen is the parasite itself.

Abnormal levels of vitamins, minerals, and liver enzymes may indicate the presence of parasitic involvement. Low serum protein and potassium levels can indicate strongyloides; low levels of vitamin B-12 may indicate fish tapeworm. Low folic acid, iron, and serum calcium may mean giardia, while low iron serum can signal the presence of hookworm. Alkaline phosphatase levels can be elevated in cases of amebiasis.

Blood tests are also used to determine malaria infection; microscopic examination will reveal parasitized red blood cells. Filaria can be diagnosed by identifying microfilariae in thick blood smears. These blood smears are best made at night, when levels of the organism are usually higher.

Available tests of the blood serum measure antibodies produced by the immune system in an attempt to fight off the parasite. These tests detect antibodies to organisms like *Entamoeba histolytica*; strongyloides; blood, liver, and lung flukes; toxocara; leishmania; *Toxoplasma gondii*; malaria; filaria; cysticerci; heartworm; and trichinella. Results of these antibody tests may not be entirely reliable with immunocompromised patients whose immune systems are so depressed they cannot produce antibodies.

Sputum Tests

A number of parasites—such as *Entamoeba histolytica,* roundworm, hookworm, strongyloides, and *Pneumocystis carinii*—can be analyzed from sputum. With roundworm, hookworm, and strongyloides, migrating larvae can produce a type of bronchitis. The resulting irritation often results in the coughing up of some of the parasites

Urine Tests

Urine testing can detect the presence of blood fluke eggs from urine sediment. Microfilariae in filarial infection can also be recovered from urine sediment. Examination of urine can frequently indicate the presence of *Trichomonas vaginalis* in both females and males. In addition, urethral discharge can reveal trichomonas in men.

Tissue Scrapings and Swabs

Perianal scrapings can be performed in cases of extraintestinal amoeba; material from the lesions is scraped and examined microscopically for evidence of the amoeba. Swabbing of the perianal area can be used to recover eggs of the pork tapeworm, beef tapeworm, and blood fluke.

The Scotch tape anal and perianal swab diagnosis is unique for the pinworm. Since the female adult worm lays her eggs around the perianal area in the early morning hours, specimens are best obtained then, before you bathe or use the bathroom. Ordinary Scotch tape—or any other brand of transparent tape—is pressed against both sides of the anal and perianal areas and then transferred to a slide for microscopic examination.

Radiologic Tests

A computerized axial tomography (CAT) scan or magnetic resonance imaging (MRI) of the brain can show brain lesions caused by toxoplasmosis and cysticercosis caused by porkworm. A CAT scan of the eye can show trapped larvae from ocular larva migrans, thereby disproving a mistaken diagnosis of retinoblastoma. A CAT scan of the liver can confirm amebic liver abscess. Common chest X-rays can detect *Pneumocystis carinii* and dog heartworm, which appears as a coin-like lesion and has sometimes been mistaken for lung cancer. In many cases, ascaris can show up in X-rays of the abdomen as outlines around intestinal gas pockets.

Aspiration

During aspiration, fluids are removed from a body cavity by suction. Rectal, liver, lung, and colon aspirations can reveal *Entamoeba histolytica*. Giardia and stronglyoides can be aspirated from the duodenum; giardia can also be aspirated from the gall bladder. Toxoplasma and leishmania can be aspirated from lymph node tissue.

Biopsy

A biopsy is removal and examination, usually microscopic, of tissue from the living body. Muscle biopsy can reveal the larvae of both the trichinella and the cysticercus of pork tapeworm. Rectal biopsy can uncover flukes, while liver biopsy is used for visceral larva migrans. Needle biopsy can show heartworm lodged in the lung while lung biopsy detects *Pneumocystis carinii*. Lymph biopsy can uncover toxoplasmosis.

Cultures

A culture is the propagation (breeding) of microorganisms or of living tissue cells in media conducive to their growth. Trichomonas can easily be cultured from vaginal samples. Worms in various life cycle stages can also be cultured. Strongyloides are among the easiest parasites to culture from stool samples. Intestinal amoeba (such as *Entamoeba histolytica*) and Acanthamoeba can be cultured. Roundworm, blood fluke, and leishmania have also been successfully cultured through various life cycle stages.

Prenatal Tests

Prenatal diagnosis of toxoplasmosis can be accomplished by analysis of amniotic fluid and fetal blood as well as by ultrasound study (sonogram) of the fetal brain. This is a very important screening that can protect your unborn child from the devastating effects of congenital toxoplasmosis, which can cause mental retardation and blindness. All pregnant women should insist upon these tests.

In France and Austria, laws require that all pregnant women be tested for toxoplasmosis. Anti-toxoplasma antibodies can be examined with a new test, the Murex single use diagnostic system (SUDS). This test provides a very fast screening for outpatient settings and is of particular value for women before and during pregnancy. (During the yearly Pap smear, all women should insist upon screening for pinworms, ascaris, and filaria, which have all been found vaginally.)

DIAGNOSTIC LABORATORIES

The following laboratories specialize in parasite testing. Your doctor can order a test for you. Some of the labs may have a physician referral service in your area. If you do not have a physician, please inquire.

Consulting Clinical and Microbiological Laboratory Inc.
1020 S.W. Taylor #855
Portland, OR 97205
(503) 222–5279

Provides ova and parasite examination, including an antigen test for giardia. A special stool culture test is offered for yeast.

Great Smokies Diagnostic Laboratory
18A Regent Park Blvd.
Asheville, NC 28806
(800) 522–4762

Specializes in multiple sample testing, including traditional microscopy techniques for rectal mucus and purged and random stool, plus high-technology techniques such as immunofluorescent staining and enzyme immunoassay for specific parasite antigens. Great Smokies provides outstanding educational materials for both the general public and the medical profession.

Lexington Professional Center
133 East 73rd Street
New York, NY 10021
(212) 988–4800

Features the Bueno-Parrish method of rectal mucus swabbing and is supervised by Hermann Bueno, M.D., and Juan Dizon, M.D.

Meridian Valley Clinical Laboratory
24030 132nd Avenue S.E.
Kent, WA 98042
(800) 234–6825

Features stool sample testing with a special giardia antigen.

Parasitic Disease Consultants Laboratory
P.O. Box 616
2177-J Flintstone Drive
Tucker, GA 30084
(404) 496–1370

Offers specialized serum tests for diagnosing malaria, schistosomiasis, strongylodiasis, trichinosis, and many other exotic parasitic infections.

Parasitology Laboratory of Washington Inc.
2141 K Street, N.W., Suite 408
Washington, DC 20037
(202) 331–0287

Features parasite stool testing under the supervision of Martin S. Wolfe, M.D. The Parasitology Lab requests you be referred by a physician. Dr. Wolfe also supervises the Travelers Medical Service of Washington at the same address. The service provides immunization, pre-travel evaluation and counseling, and post-travel diagnosis and treatment for exotic infections.

8
Treatment

*T*reatment for parasitic infection is not a "do-it-yourself" project. During treatment, many individuals experience detoxification symptoms on their road back to health. Nausea, gastrointestinal discomfort, and frequent trips to the bathroom are not uncommon. You want to be in good hands while going through this sometimes puzzling and uncomfortable process.

The question of whether to treat an asymptomatic carrier is often discussed in the medical literature. An asymptomatic carrier is an individual who is not exhibiting noticeable symptoms but is still a carrier of a parasitic infection, which could be passed on to others. Practically all researchers agree that the asymptomatic carrier should be treated because of the potential of infecting others. This is particularly important with infected children and food handlers. In some cases of parasite-based disease, the medication used to treat symptomatic individuals is not effective in the asymptomatic cyst carrier. Appropriate alternative drugs must then be utilized.

It is also believed that if one member of a family is infected, the entire family should be treated. People who live together can infect one another when making food for each other or sharing bathroom facilities. So it is a good idea to treat all household members as a matter of course.

GENERAL OBJECTIVES OF TREATMENT

Treatment of parasitic infection must be geared to *eradicating* the parasites, rather than *relieving* the symptoms of infection. If the parasites are not eradicated, the infection will continue to cause untold damage to the system. Given a proper environment, a parasite colony can flourish to sometimes fatal proportions. And so there are some symptoms of infection that should be alleviated promptly to protect the host. Parasite-induced diarrhea from amoeba, cryptosporidium, or giardia needs to be treated immediately to prevent dehydration. In immunocompromised individuals (such as those with AIDS), diarrhea can lead to severe dehydration and even death.

TREATMENT PROTOCOL

The best treatment protocol for the most commonly occurring intestinal parasites—roundworm, pinworm, and tapeworm—entails the following five steps, which should be carried out in conjunction with an experienced health-care practitioner who can guide you through the recovery process:

1. Cleansing the intestinal tract.
2. Modifying the diet.

3. Administering effective substances to eliminate the parasites.

4. Recolonizing the gastrointestinal tract with friendly bacteria.

5. Eliminating parasite risk factors from the lifestyle and environment to avoid reinfection.

Success in treatment is predicated on a number of factors. To begin with, the length of time the patient has been infected and his basic overall health are keys in determining the length of time necessary to achieve successful results. Oftentimes, repeated treatments are required for complete success, especially if the infection is of a long-standing nature. Patient cooperation, as with treatment for any illness, is crucial.

Cleansing

The first step for ridding the body of parasites naturally is to cleanse the gastrointestinal tract. Because many parasites become embedded in the intestinal wall, no type of medication can effectively reach them until the mucus and encrusted waste matter overlying the worms are softened. The intestinal cleansing process is accomplished through the use of one or more of the following natural substances: psyllium husks, agar-agar, flax seeds, comfrey root, alginate, beet root, bentonite clay, citrus pectin, and papaya extract. These substances act like a broom to sweep out the debris found in the digestive tract. (This cleansing would not be appropriate for the more exotic blood- and tissue-invasive parasites that cause malaria, trichomoniasis, toxoplasmosis, schistosomiasis, filariasis, elephantiasis, and leishmaniasis.)

Psyllium husks, flax seeds, and agar-agar are bulking agents that provide a rich source of water-soluble fiber that is without equal in removing accumulated wastes both gently and effectively. Their extremely high water-absorbing capacity allows old fecal matter that has dried on the colon wall to become lubricated and softened for normal evacuation. Because of their great swelling capacity, they are able to absorb toxins and waste materials stored in the body. The bulking agents should be taken with adequate water, so follow the specific directions for the product you use.

The laxative agents like comfrey root and beet root, and the enzymes in papaya extract, help loosen the layers of mucus on the colon wall so that they can be eliminated from the colon. It is not unusual, once you begin the cleansing process, for the body to pass strings of mucus and worms from the colon. The detoxifying agents—bentonite clay and citrus pectin—are recognized for their ability to absorb toxins from the system. Bentonite is a type of clay-like volcanic ash that has a remarkable ability to absorb many times its weight in body toxins. Citrus pectin, derived from fruit, is considered a valuable detoxifying fiber.

Most intestinal cleansing products contain one or more of the preceding ingredients. Some successful products available in most health food stores include: Nature's Way Fiber Cleanse, Sonne's No. 7 and No. 9, Colon 8 by Ion Labs, Yerba Prima Internal Cleansing Program, Nature's Most Natural Herbal System Cleanser, Perfect Seven by Agape Health Products, and The Robert Gray Intestinal Cleansing Program. Vitamin Shoppe's Colon-Enhancer can be obtained by calling (800) 223–1216. All these products contain full instructions on the labels. Be sure to read the directions carefully and take only the dosages recommended.

The Royal Flush

Colonic irrigation and home enemas can be a helpful adjunct in cleansing the colon. Colonic irrigation, sometimes called a high enema, is a procedure whereby a lukewarm water solution is irrigated into the entire length of the large intestine. The procedure, which dislodges and removes toxins over the entire length of the intestine, takes about forty-five minutes and is usually performed in a professional office. Sanitary procedures and ingredients, such as filtered water and disposable specula, are essential.

For those who prefer the do-it-yourself method, home enemas can be effective. Remember, however, that enemas reach only the lower 12½ inches of the 5½-foot colon, whereas colonic irrigation cleanses the entire length of the colon, up to the ileocecal valve.

Numerous home remedies can be added to enemas to make them more effective. Garlic's well-documented anti-parasitic properties make garlic juice enemas a beneficial treatment in cases of pinworms in children and adults. Garlic's active component, allicin, seems to be the substance that has the anti-parasitic properties.[1]

The Reverend Hanna Kroeger, a well-respected herbalist from Boulder, Colorado, suggests an enema of two mashed garlic cloves boiled in six ounces of milk and given for three consecutive nights to kill pinworms in children. Garlic enemas are also good because they support the normal acidity of the colon. Vinegar enemas (two tablespoons of apple-cider vinegar to one quart of water) are also helpful as general detoxifiers. Blackstrap molasses enemas (one tablespoon to a quart of water) will actually pull encrusted fecal matter and some parasites off the intestinal wall. Coffee enemas, used in detoxification programs, are helpful in cleansing the liver but can cause tissue weakness with prolonged use.

A word of caution when taking enemas: Use only properly filtered water, or purchase distilled water and further sterilize it by heating to a rolling boil for at least ten minutes. Sterilize the tubing and enema bag by soaking them in a diluted Clorox bath (half a teaspoon of Clorox for each gallon of water) for fifteen minutes. Rinse thoroughly with sterilized water. This procedure prevents the further introduction of water-borne parasites into your body.

Most general cleansing programs advocate the reintroduction of beneficial bacteria into the intestinal system. However, when cleansing for parasites, the protocol changes. In cases of giardia, for example, the parasites often cover complete parts of the small intestine, mechanically overcoming the normal bacterial flora. According to Great Smokies Diagnostic Laboratory, optimum bowel flora function is accomplished by destroying any parasites and pathogens.[2] So it is advisable to replenish beneficial flora after the microorganism is eradicated. Recolonizing the bowel with friendly flora is a final step, taken only after the medications used have been clinically proven successful in eradicating the problems (see page 118).

Modifying Your Diet

To date, there has been very little research regarding nutrition and parasitic-based disease in humans. Results of studies on nutritional interactions during human parasitic infections give us conflicting data. Simply put, better nutritional status helps the parasite's existence *and* improves the host's defense system. Poor nutrition will starve the parasite but will also weaken the host's immunity. There is limited definitive information for specific nutritional recommendations. Complicating variables—such as single infections being rarely observed, different parasite species affecting nutritional status in similar ways, individual parasitic organisms optimizing their own survival in several different ways while modifying their host's nutritional status, and cultural/socio-economic variables—make definitive conclusions difficult.[3]

There are studies that have shown interference with vitamin A absorption when roundworm or giardia is present. This absorption problem normalized after elimination of the worms, with or without supplementation with vitamin A.[4,5] In addition, during hookworm infestation, the severity of iron deficiency anemia has been shown to be proportionate to the number of worms present. The more severe the infestation, the more severe the deficiency. After elimination of hookworms, you should follow a high-protein diet with a daily supplementation of 50 to 100 milligrams of ferrous sulfate (taken after meals) for a minimum of three months or until hemoglobin levels return to normal.[6]

Fish tapeworms compete for vitamin B-12 in the host. After the tapeworms are eliminated from the body, it can take up to one year for B-12 levels to return to normal.[7] It is therefore important that you are patient in replenishing body supplies and are consistent in a day-to-day rebuilding of reserves. You may have been carrying around this uninvited guest for several years, so it will take some time to regenerate your system.

Despite the lack of definitive clinical human studies regarding the role of nutritional status in preventing or combatting parasite-based diseases, basic common sense and professional experience dictate certain sound nutritional practices. In my opinion, the cleansing program should be accompanied by a therapeutic diet that supports the host and starves the parasite. Diet strongly influences the intestinal environment. A diet high in simple carbohydrates like sugar, white flour, and processed foods can provide the ideal feeding ground for worms. Even so-called "natural sweets"—honey, barley malt, fruit, fruit juice sweeteners and concentrates—taken in excess can provide instant food for your internal hitchhikers. Fiber-deficient foods may have initially precipitated a breeding ground for parasites. These foods require more time to pass through the alimentary system. A sluggish transit time allows more food to decay and putrefy, thus producing stagnation in the colon and an inviting environment for parasites.

A Supportive Therapeutic Diet

In my fifteen years of experience with clients, I have found that a diet composed of 25 percent fat, 25 percent protein, and 50 percent complex carbohydrates works well for parasite-ridden bodies. The diet must have sufficient unprocessed oils (at least one to two tablespoons daily) from 100 percent expeller pressed safflower, sesame, flax, and canola oils. These oils lubricate the gastrointestinal tract and serve as a carrier for fat-soluble vitamin A. It appears that of all vitamins and minerals, vitamin A best increases resistance to tissue penetration by parasite larvae.[8] Animals fed diets deficient in vitamin A have shown an increase in tissue penetration by parasitic larvae[9,10]. Foods rich in vitamin A such as cooked carrots, squash, sweet potatoes, yams, and greens should, therefore, be amply included in the diet.

Eating sufficient, properly cooked protein (meat, fish, chicken, eggs) is vital to a supportive therapeutic diet. Protein provides the amino-acid building blocks necessary to strengthen tissues and enhance immunity. Studies show that children who suffer from malnutrition caused by roundworms benefit from increased protein intake.[11] Thus, a moderately-high-protein diet of well-cooked turkey, chicken, fish, and lamb that is easily digested, with lots of cooked vegetables, stews, and soups, may be the best therapeutic diet. For vegetarians, Multiminophan, a multiple source of natural free-form essential amino acids, can be used as a protein supplement. Multiminophan is available from Uni Key Health Systems (800–888–4353), a mail order company that specializes in parasite-related health products.

Vegetarians and others who depend upon protein sources such as beans, nuts, seeds, peas, and legumes will need to restrict their intake of such foods. These high-fiber foods, in the presence of parasitic infections, cause flatulence and irritate the gastrointestinal tract. This further prevents the absorption of nutrients. However, because research has shown that a high-fiber diet helps prevent giardiasis,[12] a water-soluble fiber supplement that is gentler to the gastrointestinal tract is recommended. Less irritating fiber supplements include psyllium seed husks, rice bran, and oat bran.

Soy products such as tofu and tempeh can be included in moderation, i.e., not more than once or twice a week. Soy products leave an alkaline residue in the system, and it has been my experience that in parasite diet therapy, the system needs to be more acidic on a cellular level. An overly alkaline condition in the gastrointestinal tract provides a favorable environment for protozoans and worms.[13] Because several parasites, like roundworm and giardia, precipitate secondary lactose intolerances that sometimes persist after elimination of the parasites, limiting or completely avoiding dairy products during and after treatment may be necessary. Because of the damaged intestinal villi, giardia can also produce gluten intolerance—the inability to digest the protein portion of wheat and rye and, to a lesser degree, oats and barley. With any protozoan infection that can damage the intestinal villi, it is always a good idea to reduce the intake of grains (with the exception of gluten-free rice and millet).

Heavy intake of raw fruits and vegetables should be greatly curtailed, and cold or iced foods and drinks should be avoided. These foods cause the intestines to contract, thereby holding in toxins rather than releasing them. For the therapeutic parasite control diet, cook most fruits and vegetables so they will be more easily digested and more soothing to the intestinal tract. Raw vegetable and fruit juices are not suggested at this time.

A well-balanced, supportive eating program is essential because malabsorption often occurs from parasitic damage to the intestine. Especially common in parasite infections is decreased absorption of fats and proteins and decreased absorption of vitamins, including beta-carotene, vitamin A, folic acid, and vitamin B-12.[14] A graphic example of this nutritional interaction between host and parasite can be seen in the case of the fish tapeworm. The adult tapeworm is "able to obtain as much as 75% to 100% of a physiological dose of vitamin B-12 before the vitamin is absorbed by the mucosa."[15]

Eating the right foods, however, may not be enough to ensure proper nutritional support. Many people lack an adequate supply of the digestive enzymes that are needed to release the nutrients contained in foods. Even with a good diet, enzyme deficiencies can lead to nutritional deficiencies and weakened resistance.

Enzyme deficiencies also lead to incompletely digested foods that can putrefy or ferment in the intestines, creating an environment that is ripe for parasites. Concentrated plant enzymes from aspergillus (a fungal-type microorganism used in the fermentation of miso and soy sauce) can be used as a dietary supplement to help correct the underlying conditions that favor parasitic infections. One commercial preparation I recommend for this purpose is Vitase by Avail Corporation; it helps to digest dietary proteins, carbohydrates, fats, sugars, and fiber.

Administering Anti-Parasitic Substances

Besides the basic diet recommendations, there are special foods that have time-tested anti-parasitic properties. Among these are fresh pineapple and papaya, which contain high amounts of natural protein-digesting enzymes like bromelain and papain and have long been used by natives of Mexico to cure worm infestations. Because of the sugar content of these fruits, it may be better to take them in supplement form where the extracts are often combined with pepsin and hydrochloric acid, which aid not only in food digestion but in digestion of the parasites. In cases of giardia, digestive enzyme supplements containing ox bile or bile salts should be avoided, as recent research reports that bile sparks the growth of giardia and bile salt is eagerly devoured by the parasite.[16]

Pomegranate juice, up to four glasses per day, available in health food stores or made at home with your juicer, is effective against tapeworm infection. In Mexico, papaya seeds are used for their parasite-eliminating powers. Used in salad dressings, their peppery taste can add a little zip. Finely ground pumpkin seeds (one-fourth to half a cup) made into a porridge can be taken on a daily basis to eliminate many varieties of worms. Native Americans often chewed pumpkin seeds as an effective deworming agent (vermifuge). Garlic has been used since ancient times as a vermifuge. Two cloves of raw garlic per day used in food preparation can be effective against roundworms, pinworms, tapeworms, and hookworms in both humans and animals. Onions, carrot tops, radish roots, kelp, raw cabbage, ground almonds, blackberries, pumpkin, sauerkraut, and fig extract also have anti-parasitic qualities.

Herbal Cures

Many effective herbs have been used by both Eastern and Western cultures to kill and expel parasites and worms. Some of the most effective include garlic, black walnut bark (including the kernel and green hull), butternut root bark, pinkroot, goldenseal, wormwood, sage, clove, tansy, fennel, thyme, cranberry powder, and male fern. Some of these herbs, like fennel, thyme, sage, and garlic, can be used for seasonings in everyday cooking. Others are commonly available at health food stores in capsules, powders, and tinctures. Directions for use can be found on product bottles. Most herbal formulas on the market are usually taken before meals (presumably to immobilize the parasite before food is ingested) and sometimes before bedtime for ten days to two weeks.

Folklore instructions suggest that any course of treatment for worms should begin around the full moon when the parasites supposedly become more active in the system. When beginning herbal treatments, it is a good idea to start with low doses for a few days to assure that there are no individual sensitivities. After the full course of treatment, allow the body to cleanse itself naturally before attacking the next reproductive cycle of internal boarders with another course of herbs.

Over the years, I have researched, experimented with, and written about various products. My clients and readers have reported very satisfactory results with several natural preparations. All the preparations mentioned in the following paragraphs can be ordered by calling Uni

Key Health Systems at (800) 888–4353. One such product, Paratox 11, is effective against the larger parasites or worms. This product contains ingredients such as black walnut, senna blend, pinkroot, slippery elm, and garlic. The primary ingredient—black walnut—kills many types of worms. The Chinese have used it for centuries to kill tapeworm. Pinkroot, also known as Indian pink, was used by Native Americans because of its remarkable cure rate for intestinal worms, especially roundworms. The other ingredients are both laxative and cleansing to the body. Paratox 11 can be taken for a period of two weeks, with two to four capsules taken with a large glass of warm water at least twenty minutes before each meal. Then discontinue use for two weeks. Repeat the cycle up to four times to assure that all larvae are eliminated and parasite testing results are negative.

A product designed for microscopic parasites (Protozoa) is Paratox 22, a combination of grapefruit seed extract, garlic, slippery elm, and cranberry concentrate. This blend of ingredients penetrates the mucosal lining of the gastrointestinal tract where both Protozoa and fungus reside. Slippery elm helps soothe gastrointestinal irritation, while cranberry concentrate is rich in organic acids (citric, malic, quinic, and benzoic) that aid in the digestion of the Protozoa. Paratox 22 is taken in the same way as Paratox 11 (two to four capsules before each meal, two weeks on, two weeks off, repeated up to four times).

Two other beneficial remedies are Artemisia Annua Extract, a relative of American wormwood, and Paracan-MYC. Artemisia Annua Extract exhibits strong anti-malarial properties as well as effectiveness against worms and various parasites. This herbal product crosses the gut wall and has anti-parasitic effects throughout the entire system. Paracan-MYC is derived from grapefruit seed and pulp. Grapefruit seed extract has been shown to help elimi-

nate Protozoa and fungus on contact. One to three capsules of Paracan-MYC are taken two times a day.

Once parasites and worms are eliminated, I usually
recommend that my clients take capsules of Zymex II, a
preparation by Standard Process Labs for the digestion of
any remaining larvae and eggs in the intestine. Zymex II
is a combination of proteolytic enzymes from almond
flour, fig powder, papain, bromelain, lipase, cellulase,
and amylase. Two capsules should be taken between
meals two to three times daily.

Homeopathic Remedies

There are also several homeopathic remedies for parasitic
infections. Homeopathy, a healing process that has been
practiced in Europe for almost 200 years, is based upon the
premise that "like cures like." Homeopaths believe that any
substance capable of inducing symptoms in a healthy individual will, in minute amounts, remove those same symptoms in a diseased person. Among homeopathic remedies
for parasite infection are the following:

Remedy	Parasite or condition
Chelidonium	liver flukes
Chenopodium	hookworm/roundworm
Cina	pinworm
Felix mas	tapeworm
Santoninum	roundworm/threadworm

Other homeopathic remedies that are anti-parasitic
include the tissue cell salts sodium phosphate and calcium
phosphate. The cell salt natrum sulphate is a well-respected systemic tonic for parasitic conditions.

As a temporary treatment for nausea resulting from

amoeba and giardia infection, the homeopathic 6x potency of ipecacuanha can be used. While the full-strength ipecac syrup is used to induce vomiting, the homeopathic dilution causes no adverse reaction and is quite successful in alleviating nausea. It is best that homeopathic remedies be selected and used under the guidance of a qualified homeopathic physician or naturopath.

Effective Drugs

Many effective drugs are used against parasitic infections. In the appendix, I have included a protocol for physician reference from *The Medical Letter on Drugs and Therapeutics*. As the *Medical Letter* states:

> In every case, the need for treatment must be weighed against the toxicity of the drug. A decision to withhold therapy may often be correct, particularly when the drugs can cause severe adverse effects.[17]

The *Medical Letter* includes a very comprehensive listing of the adverse effects of some anti-parasitic drugs. Metronidazole (Flagyl), for example, used in the treatment of giardiasis, amebiasis, and trichomoniasis, can cause nausea, headaches, disorientation, and a metallic taste in the mouth. In addition, Flagyl encourages yeast growth, thereby wreaking more havoc on an already compromised immune system. Parasite expert Dr. Louis Parrish writes in the *Townsend Newsletter* with regard to parasites that many physicians are under the misconception that:

> . . . treatment with a single course of metronidazole (Flagyl) is 90% effective. The facts: 25 years ago this may have been true, but the protozoa rapidly become

resistant. Today the single course cure rate is less than 5%. Furthermore, approximately half of the patients treated with metronidazole complain of side effects, and 10% flatly refuse to take it ever again.[18]

In light of this, some physicians are choosing to use more natural remedies that have proven to be safer and just as effective. Patients report good success with these remedies and minimal side effects.

Recolonization of the Intestinal Tract

Reintroduction of friendly bacteria in the intestinal tract following the complete eradication of foreign visitors is the final step in natural treatment methods. These friendly flora help detoxify noxious substances, maintain proper pH, and act as natural antibiotics against infectious bacteria. This, along with continuation of proper diet and lifestyle habits, can protect the body against future invasions.

The bacteria strains I have found most helpful in recolonizing the bowel include *Lactobacillus acidophilus*, *Lactobacillus bulgaris*, *Lactobacillus bifidus*, and *Streptococcus faeceum*. Many people need one or a combination of all four to repopulate the intestinal tract. There are many high-quality, hypoallergenic acidophilus-type formulations on the market. My patients have reported good results using Aqua Flora, a homeopathic anti-yeast liquid formula that reduces yeast overgrowth and allows beneficial bacteria to regenerate. Aqua Flora is available through Uni Key Health Systems at (800) 888–4353.

Another helpful product is Inner Ecology by Avail; it contains four strains of friendly bacteria to recolonize the intestine, and includes fructo-oligosaccharides (FOS). FOS, a naturally occurring carbohydrate found in Jerusalem artichoke and other foods, stimulates the growth of beneficial bacteria up to ten-fold, according to studies.[19] Aqua Flora and Inner Ecology are available through Uni Key Health Systems at (800) 888–4353.

Whatever products you consider, check your local health food stores and read the labels carefully. Friendly flora is available in liquid, powder, and pill forms. Whichever form you select, be sure to follow the manufacturer's instructions. More is not necessarily better. Daily use is good insurance against further infestation and also aids in maintaining a healthy immune system.

Elimination of Parasite Risk Factors

This part of the treatment program is truly do-it-yourself because I have no straightforward answers. Only you can uncover the reason(s) you played host to parasites in the first place. Take a look back at Chapter Six and review the questionnaire once again. Do you frequently travel to exotic foreign locales and live like the natives? Are you a sushi lover? Do you like your meat extra rare? Are you in the habit of kissing your dog? Does your water come from a natural mountain spring?

Take responsibility for changing lifestyle, food, and environmental habits that put you in harm's way. The next chapter offers very specific guidelines to assist you in this process.

9
Prevention

*T*his is the most important chapter in the book. Since parasites are difficult to find, and often more difficult to treat, the best solution is to prevent them in the first place. Since some of them, like giardia, are fast becoming a fact of life, we will have to learn to live with them by strengthening our resistance to them. Parasites are opportunistic critters. Any flaw or weakness in our defense system is an open invitation to invasion.

Our best line of defense against parasitic infection is a strong, healthy immune system. But our immune systems have taken a beating in the past few decades. Every year, 2.6 billion pounds of pesticides are used in the United States, mostly on food crops. The food we eat, instead of nourishing our bodies, challenges our immune systems with residues from these pesticides. Unless we take the time and care involved to clean our fresh fruits and vegetables as outlined later in this chapter, these very healthful foods can be the vehicle by which parasites enter our bodies, along with chemical and pesticide residues.

The ground water supplies in over half the states in this country have been contaminated with pesticides from run-off. And, as discussed in Chapter Four, many municipal water supplies are antiquated and have become breeding grounds of giardia, bacteria, viruses, lead, and other contaminants. Even the air we breathe contains pollutants that challenge our immune systems. Each challenge to the immune system stimulates it into action. Parasites, as foreign invaders, also activate the immune response. As the parasites continue their invasion unchecked, the damage they cause to the body's vital systems, including the gastrointestinal and nervous systems, creates further stress on an already weakened immune system. This continual assault and damage eventually leads to immune system exhaustion.

Supporting our immune systems with foods rich in vitamins C, E, and beta-carotene and the minerals zinc and selenium is a good first line of defense against parasitic infection. Additional supplementation with these vitamins and minerals and with herbs like echinacea, ginseng, and astragalus is good insurance for a healthy immune system. These vitamins, minerals, and herbs have been shown in numerous studies to enhance and support immunity.

Since most parasites enter the body orally, one of the body's best defenses against them is our stomach acid. Very few pathogenic microorganisms can survive the hydrochloric acid in a healthy stomach. However, numerous factors lead to a lack of hydrochloric acid in the body:

- An overgrowth of *Candida albicans* can damage the cells that produce hydrochloric acid. A course of antibiotics can often result in an overgrowth of *Candida albicans*, leaving one of our body's best defenses against parasites severely weakened.

- Recent research has shown that people with type A blood have a genetic predisposition to a condition known as achlorhydria, whereby the body does not produce enough hydrochloric acid.

- Lead, one of the more toxic heavy metals widely distributed in our environment, binds the hydrochloric acid in our stomachs, making it unavailable for digestion.

Like the prevention of other major health problems, the prevention of parasitic infections must begin with the awareness that we are all at risk, even if we never travel outside the United States. By following the guidelines in this chapter in regard to personal and household hygiene, travel, sexual practices, food and water, day-care and school sanitation, household pets, and eating out, you can protect yourself and your family. I have put these guidelines into an outline form for easy reading and reference. At first they may seem overwhelming to some people. But the good news is that many of the common avenues of transmission are within our control. Armed with the proper information and education regarding our current-day environment, hygiene, sanitation, and food, we *can* overcome.

PERSONAL HYGIENE

We often overlook the importance of personal hygiene. Here's a reminder.

- *Always* wash your hands prior to eating.
- Make sure to wash your hands with soap and water

after going to the bathroom, changing the baby's diaper, or handling your pets.

- Be sure to keep fingernails short and scrub under them. (A nail brush kept in the bathroom is a good idea.)
- Don't sit on a bare toilet seat without first wiping it or protecting it with toilet paper. Better still, squat. Pinworm eggs and trichomonas can lurk under toilet seats. Trichomonas can also be spread through mud baths, water baths, and sauna benches.
- Don't use tap water to clean contact lenses. Distilled water can also be contaminated, so buy sterilized lens preparations for all cleansing and disinfecting purposes. Make sure to remove contact lenses before swimming.
- Don't walk barefoot, especially in warm, moist, sandy soil.
- If you travel frequently, eat out on a regular basis, have pets, or live in a mountainous region of the country, have a complete parasite examination at least twice a year. The most accurate diagnosis comes from a combination of purged stool and rectal mucous exam. (See Chapter Seven.)

INFANT AND CHILD CARE

Healthful habits should be practiced and taught at the earliest stages of childhood.

- Breast-feed your baby as long as you can. Human milk has anti-protozoan properties, which provide antibodies that fight against amoeba and giardia.
- Keep toddlers away from puppies and kittens that have not been regularly dewormed.

- Be sure your child routinely washes after contact with household pets. With infants, the task is *your* responsibility.
- It's a good idea to prevent toddlers from kissing household pets or being licked by them.
- Do not allow children to eat dirt.
- Do not allow children to play in yards, playgrounds, or sandboxes in which animals are allowed to roam loose.
- Clean children's bedrooms with a damp mop or vacuum to avoid stirring up possibly infested dust.
- Sanitize all toilet seats and bowls, but particularly those used by children, with a mild Clorox solution. Clean the undersurface of the seat.
- Clean children's toys with mild, soapy water.
- Keep children's fingernails short and clean.

Procedures for an Infected Child

Children who have pinworms should follow these additional preventive measures to avoid the spread and reinfection among other family members. These tips come from Leo Litter, M.D., a pediatrician in West Hartford, Connecticut:

- Bathe daily.
- Use one washcloth and towel for the face and hands, another for baths.
- Scrub hands thoroughly after bathroom use and before each meal.
- Wear close-fitting underpants at all times (under sleeping garments, too).

- Do not share a bed.

Procedures for an Infected Child's Caregivers

Mom and Dad can help by instituting these additional measures:

- Launder bedclothing and personal clothing of the infected person daily.
- Keep toothbrushes in containers (thus avoiding exposure to bathroom dust that transmits pinworms).
- Scrub toilet seats daily.
- Clean and vacuum daily (to remove eggs along with the dirt).
- Keep all rooms—bedrooms, especially—well aired.
- As frequently as practical, superheat the home to 95°F for a day. Dr. Litter suggests this is the most effective way to kill embryos in the eggs. He suggests the children's room be heated to 95°F for just a day, preferably on a weekend when the family members are out.

WATER USAGE

Avoid water-borne disease by paying careful attention to what you drink.

- Have your tap water tested. The EPA Safe Drinking Water Hotline can tell you who to contact. In Alaska and Washington D.C., call (202) 382–5533; elsewhere, call (800) 426–4791 between 8:30 A.M. and 4:30 P.M. EST.
- Drink only filtered water. To filter microorganism cysts

effectively, a fine pore filter of not more than three microns is necessary. In a study conducted at Colorado State University, Fort Collins, Colorado, the following four filters blocked Giardia cysts from tap water: Royal Doulton (model F 303), Seagul IV (model X1F), Micro Twin (model 10 TOBC), and Everpure (model QC4). Frequent changing of the filter assures consistently uncontaminated water.

Other water treatment systems that help block parasites include Pure Water Aquathin, Multi-Pure, and Nature's Spring. A microfiltration system specifically designed to block microorganisms is also available through Amway.

- If you hike, camp, ski, or swim, never drink out of brooks, reservoirs, ponds, streams, or lakes no matter how pristine or remote they may seem. Water must be boiled or filtered.

- If backpacking, camping out, or traveling in mountainous regions of the United States or abroad, invest in a portable water filter designed to filter out giardia cysts. A fine pore filter of not more than three microns is desirable. Charcoal filters must contain a fine pore filter. Portable drinking-water filters that remove giardia include General Ecology First Need, and the Timberline Filter; these filters can be purchased at outdoor and camping stores. The Katadyn is one of the best portable pocket filters on the market and has been used by the North Atlantic Treaty Organization (NATO). It can be purchased from Provisions Unlimited, P.O. Box 456, Oakland, Maine 04963. It weighs about twenty-three ounces and so is fairly lightweight as well as extremely efficient with a pore filter of two microns. The other filters can be purchased at outdoor and camping stores.

FOOD HANDLING

Parasite infection can be avoided by treating all foods in a special cleansing bath. To remove parasites as well as sprays, fungi, and bacteria from food, soak all meat, fish, lamb, eggs, vegetables, and fruit thoroughly according to the following procedure:

1. Use half a teaspoon of Clorox to one gallon of water, obtained from your usual source. (To ensure that you are using the proper preparation, Dr. Hazel Parcells recommends that you use only the brand-name bleach Clorox.) Make sure to be careful when using bleach. At full strength, it is a powerful chemical.

2. Place the foods to be treated into the bath according to the following chart. Make a separate bath for each grouping.

Food Group	Treatment Time
Leafy vegetables	15 minutes
Root vegetables, thick-skinned vegetables, fibrous vegetables	30 minutes
Thin-skinned berries, peaches, apricots, plums	15 minutes
Thick-skinned fruits such as apples, citrus, bananas	30 minutes
Chicken, fish, meats, eggs (Each protein food should be treated in its own bath.)	20 minutes

Note: Meats can be thawed in a Clorox bath. The timing is about twenty minutes for a weight between two and five pounds. Frozen turkey or chicken should remain in the Clorox bath until thawed. Ground meats, of course, cannot be treated this way.

---

3. Remove foods from the Clorox bath and place into clear water for ten minutes. This is the rinse bath. Finish cleaning, dry all foods thoroughly, and store.

- If you choose not to use Clorox, freeze fish at –18°C for at least forty-eight hours to kill larvae. Freeze beef and pork at –20°C for at least twenty-four hours to kill larvae.

- To ensure 100 percent parasite-proof food, consider investing in cookware by Royal Prestige. Food is cooked by the minimum moisture method at 180°F—the temperature that kills germs, bacteria, and parasites, not vitamins and minerals. Royal Prestige is available through Uni Key, which may be contacted at (800) 888–4353.

- When cooking meat in a conventional oven, always set the temperature to at least 325°F. The use of a meat thermometer is suggested when cooking in conventional ovens, and the internal temperature should be checked in several places. Beef should be cooked to an internal temperature of at least 160°F; lamb, veal, and pork to 170°F. Check for doneness always—i.e., no pink—especially in the center.

- When cooking meat or fish in a microwave oven, be aware that microwaves heat unevenly. Be sure to check the internal temperature in many different places. Fish must be heated to an internal temperature of 140°F for at least five minutes.

- In conventional ovens, cook fish until it's flaky and white. Bake at 400°F, eight to ten minutes per inch of thickness.

- It is best to buy your seafood from established dealers rather than from roadside stands or trucks.

- Use a mild bleach solution to clean all cooking utensils, cutting boards (particularly if they are wooden where bacteria can easily be trapped), or surfaces that have come in contact with uncooked foods.

- Avoid the habit of sampling dishes like sausage and gefilte fish before they are thoroughly cooked.

- Try to eat Pacific salmon and/or Pacific rockfish (red snapper) that has been commercially blast-frozen. If you eat sushi, avoid any that has been made from Pacific salmon and Pacific rockfish. These are known to contain parasites. Ask that your fish market carry blast-frozen fish.

- Unless you are an experienced sushi chef, it is best not to prepare raw fish dishes like sushi and sashimi at home. Experienced chefs are highly trained to know which fish species can be infected, and they can spot larvae.

- A food safety hotline sponsored by the Alliance for Food and Fibers Food Safety Information is available. Call (800) 266–0200 with your questions.

- Maintain a balanced diet with moderate amounts of protein, high fiber, natural complex carbohydrates, such as beans, starchy root vegetables, and a variety of whole grains. Use lots of garlic in cooking. Snack on pumpkin seeds. Remember that parasites thrive on sweets and simple carbohydrates, so limit even natural sources of sugar from fruit and fruit juice, for example, to two or three portions a day. Natural oils in the form of unprocessed, expeller pressed safflower, sunflower, corn, flax, and sesame can strengthen the immune system by fortifying the cell membrane walls. Refer to *Beyond Pritikin* (see page 159) for more information on the importance of essential fat in the diet for general overall health. (The book also contains menu ideas, shopping lists, food portion guides, and recipes for maintaining good health.)

- Use an unrefined natural sea salt in cooking. Salt has an antiseptic effect on body tissues.
- When eating out, skip the salad bars. Order only well-cooked food.

TRAVEL ARRANGEMENTS

The enormous increase in worldwide travel may expose tourists to rare diseases. Pre-travel information on food, water, and other hygienic practices is recommended and can be obtained from The Traveler's Medical Service of Washington, D.C., at (202) 466–8109.

- When planning a trip abroad, be sensible and prepare well in advance. Contact the Traveler's Health Section of the Centers for Disease Control in Atlanta at (404) 629–3311 to obtain guides to regional diseases in the areas where you will be traveling.
- When traveling abroad or in mountainous regions of the United States where giardia thrives, take along your portable water filter or drink only from reliable bottled water sources. Eat only cooked or peeled fruits and vegetables. Avoid ice cubes in your drinks; they most likely have been made from tap water. Do not brush your teeth with tap water.
- Avoid regional foods and special dishes that include raw, pickled, smoked, or dried fish, crabs, and crayfish. All beef and lamb should be thoroughly cooked.
- Consider taking along Pepto-Bismol as a diarrhea pre-

ventative. Take two ounces four times daily or one to two tablets four times a day for every day of travel. Freeze-dried acidophilus (which doesn't need refrigeration) is a beneficial intestinal bacteria that, taken before each meal, can help prevent "Traveler's Diarrhea" or "Montezuma's Revenge."

- Bentonite, a clay-like liquid found in most health food stores, is a good natural parasite preventative. When taken in the morning and evening (at least one tablespoon each time) it has been known to protect travelers from disease by absorbing poisons in the intestinal tract and flushing them out of the system. My clients who are prone to diarrhea when they travel no longer are stricken after taking bentonite along.

- Avoid swimming in freshwater lakes.

- If you are sleeping in a tent in tropical areas, sleep under well-screened netting. Do not wear perfumes or after-shaves; they attract mosquitoes. Use insect repellent only.

- When traveling in the tropics, Africa, Asia, or the Middle East, stay covered up. Wear long sleeves and long pants. Be particularly careful at night. The *Anopheles* mosquito that carries malaria comes out between dusk and dawn. You might also, in tropical climates, consider taking vitamin B-1 (about 50 to 100 milligrams per day) or brewer's yeast tablets (at least three tablets three times per day) to help naturally repel both fleas and mosquitoes from your body.

SEXUAL PRACTICES

Prevention of sexually transmitted parasitic disease depends on practicing safe sex and avoiding certain sexual practices.

- Regardless of sexual preference, wear condoms when engaging in sexual intercourse.
- Gay men should avoid playing with "toys" that may contain contaminated fecal matter.
- Avoid oral-anal sex to prevent transmission of trichomonas, pinworms, ascaris, *Entamoeba histolytica*, giardia, and strongyloides.
- Gay men should use a condom when engaging in any form of sexual contact.

ANIMAL CARE

Since household pets are nearly universally infected with certain parasites, every pet can be a source of infection.

- Be a "pooper scooper." Don't allow your dogs and cats to defecate on lawns and playgrounds, or in sandboxes. Collect and discard your animal's droppings. Feces should be burned or flushed whenever possible.
- Empty the kitty litter box daily. Gloves should be worn for this task. Feces should be burned or flushed down the toilet. Litter boxes should be cleaned frequently and disinfected with boiling water and a mild bleach solution. Pregnant women and immunocompromised patients in particular should wear disposable gloves and mask or, better still, relegate this responsibility to someone else.
- Keep animals outside the home if toddlers are in the house.
- Deworm all puppies and kittens on a regular basis. Some veterinarians suggest to begin at three and six

weeks of age and continue with routine deworming every six months. Consult with your local veterinarian.

- Routinely check your animal's stool for worms yourself and then report to your vet.

- Have your veterinarian check for roundworm and tapeworm infections if the animal shows signs of illness or is rubbing its anus against the carpet or floor. Pumpkin-seed-like particles found near the animal or where it has roamed are a sign of dog tapeworm.

- Consider keeping cats indoors to prevent their access to rodents and birds. They should be fed canned or dry cat food and only cooked, not raw, meat.

- Buy flea collars, or apply topical insecticides to dogs and cats to kill all fleas. A periodic flea bath may be necessary for thorough eradication.

- For a more natural approach, you might try adding fennel, rosemary, rue, or garlic to the animal's food to help repel fleas from the inside out. Garlic and yeast wafers are parasite- and flea-proof foods for your animals. Regularly disinfect your animal's food dish and water bowl with mild soapy water, then a diluted Clorox solution.

- To protect children playing in dirt from inadvertently ingesting soil contaminated with toxocara eggs, turn backyard soil under if your animal plays outside.

- Keep sandboxes covered.

- Provide your pet with filtered drinking water in a regularly cleaned container.

- Regularly brush and clean pets outdoors.

- Make sure all kitchen or dining room areas designed for food preparation or eating—i.e., counter tops, tables, refrigerator, dining room table—are strictly off-limits to your pets.

ON THE JOB

Many job-related activities can be a source of parasitic infection. Those whose jobs take them to developing countries for long periods of time are especially at risk.

- Overseas consultants, laborers, diplomats, and missionaries, as well as family members who accompany them, should be periodically examined with a complete blood count, liver function tests, and purged stool examination.
- All veterinary personnel, kennel workers, pet shop employees, animal trainers, sanitation workers, gardeners, zoo personnel, and cattle feedlot workers should be regularly checked for animal-transmitted infections.
- Check to see that your child's day-care center maintains good hygiene practices. All employees should routinely wash hands and scrub under the fingernails after using the bathroom and changing diapers. Children should be instructed in these good hygiene practices, too. Toys and water faucets should be cleaned daily. Diaper changing should be relegated to one area, which should be cleaned after each changing with a soapy water solution. Children suffering from diarrhea should be kept at home.
- Every food handler in restaurants, hotels, and school or workplace cafeterias should be required to undergo stool testing. (We should all work to see that legislation for mandatory stool testing is enacted.)

AT HOME

On the home front, there are often unsuspected risks for parasite infection which need closer scrutiny.

- Keep the home environment rodent-free to avoid exposure to rat tapeworm.
- In suburban and rural settings, watch out for raccoons. Their feces can be deposited in soil and objects that find their way into children's mouths. Raccoons carry roundworms, and over half may be infected. The Veterinary Medical Association has warned about the potential roundworm threat particularly, because small children chew and suck on objects that may be contaminated by raccoon feces in suburban neighborhoods.
- When employing a nanny, maid, or housekeeper, first screen her by using the questionnaire in Chapter Six. Use your judgment if you feel further medical testing is necessary. This is particularly important if this person is going to be preparing food for you and your family.

FOR WOMEN ONLY

Women, because of their anatomical design, need to take special preventative measures.

- After urinating, wipe from front to back.
- When you have your yearly Pap smear, have the lab look for possible cervical pinworms and roundworms if you suspect a problem in the vaginal area or if you have frequent sexual relations with multiple partners.
- Be screened for toxoplasmosis if you are pregnant or attempting pregnancy.

- If pregnant, limit your exposure to cats. If possible, have someone else be caretaker of the household cat. Keep your pet away from your food, and, in any event, have the cat checked for *Toxoplasma gondii*. Avoid undercooked meat.

Protecting you and your family from parasites involves a multifaceted approach. Old-fashioned common sense coupled with a heightened awareness and understanding of the methods of transmission and sources of potential infection are key factors in prevention. Our bodies are bombarded on a daily basis with a multitude of disease-producing bacteria, viruses, and allergens. The body's natural defender, our immune system, prevents us from "catching" germs and becoming host to every passing microbe.

I am reminded of the Ayurvedic (Indian) proverb that states, "If the field is barren, the seed, howsoever potent, may not be able to germinate." In other words, parasites cannot infect a healthy body if the environment isn't conducive to them. Andreas Marx, a doctor of oriental medicine, said it best when he linked disease to "an imbalance of the body's terrain (pH, oxidation factor, and mineral balance)." We can stay healthy by nourishing our bodies with healthy food; supplementing our diets with immune-enhancing vitamins, minerals, and herbs; and by eliminating parasite risk factors from our environment.

10
Closing Comments

arasitic infections are a reality in the United States today. Our water, food, pets, restaurants, and daycare centers are all potential sources of infection. Because there is sometimes no effective course of action for the treatment of these parasite-based disorders, prevention is most important. Trichinosis, for example, can be prevented by cooking meat to 170°F, but there is no therapy that has proven effective for treating this infection.[1] The animal-transmitted infection visceral larva migrans occurs most commonly in children who have pets or who play in areas that are frequented by dogs and cats. And since 60 percent of this country's 85 million households have a pet dog or cat, that puts literally millions of our children at risk. We can reduce this risk by following the guidelines in Chapter Nine, but there is no effective treatment for the respiratory and eye problems resulting from a visceral larva migrans infection.

But there is no need to become paranoid. We just need to become more responsible and conscious of a problem that many of us are not aware even exists. Parasites can only persist when they have a suitable environment. Diets high in sugars, refined carbohydrates, and fiber-depleted processed foods, and immune systems that have been weakened by these diets and by other environmental consequences of modern-day living, provide the ideal feeding ground for parasites. The problem is not so much "out there" as it is within our bodies.

On a national level, a great deal of energy and effort are directed toward educating the public regarding preventative measures for today's most threatening diseases—heart disease, cancer, AIDS. And more and more people are making lifestyle changes as public health education makes them aware of the risk factors related to these diseases—poor diet, environmental pollution, lack of exercise, smoking, drug and alcohol abuse, etc.

Heart disease, cancer, AIDS . . . these are not silent epidemics. The parasite problem, however, *is* a silent epidemic. There is a dangerous misconception that parasitic infections occur only in tropical areas or among the poor who live in unsanitary conditions. This misconception has resulted in a lack of awareness of the risk factors and symptoms associated with this insidious public health threat in America today. Furthermore, American doctors and other medical professionals have had so little training or experience with parasitic diseases that they are not alert to clinical symptoms. One of the most up-to-date clinical parasitology textbooks concludes:

> The most important element in diagnosing a parasitic infection is often the physician's suspicion that a parasite may be involved—a possibility that is too often overlooked.[2]

The physician's lack of suspicion and concurrent underdiagnosis has left the public totally unaware of the scope of the parasite problem.

Making the matter even more complicated, the random stool examination—the standard method of detection used by most physicians who do routinely check for parasites—has proven to be insufficient and unreliable. Unfortunately, based upon false negative results from inadequate testing procedures, most physicians rule out parasites as an underlying cause of disease. Since many symptoms of these infections are often non-specific and mimic other, more-recognizable diseases, the condition is then misdiagnosed and health problems persist for months and sometimes even years before the real culprit is identified.

The study of parasitology in medical schools must be taken out of the departments of tropical diseases, because parasites are not just tropical any more. All physicians, regardless of field of speciality, should be required to take basic courses in parasitology so that they suspect parasite-based disease when it is present and know how to effectively diagnosis it, treat it, and prevent its recurrence. We all must become responsible for the quality and safety of the food we eat and water we drink, for the way we handle our pets, for protecting ourselves when traveling, and for demanding appropriate medical testing and care when we suspect the possibility of parasitic infection.

Today, we are all susceptible to a wide array of parasite-related illness, ranging from rather common infections to rare disease manifestations. Our expanded travel opportunities and sanitation breakdowns on the homeland have exposed us to a surprising number of uninvited guests. *Guess What Came to Dinner* provides some of the solutions to the chronic ill health that Americans in the 1990s are experiencing.

Glossary

AIDS. Acquired immune deficiency syndrome. A disease of the body's infection-fighting system, thought to be caused by the HTLV-3 virus.

Acanthamoeba keratitis. A type of amoeba that causes corneal inflammation.

Alveoli. Air sacs in the lungs.

Amebiasis. An infection caused by internal animal parasites called amoebas.

Amoeba. Any of the protozoans of the genus *Amoeba* having an indefinite changeable form.

Anopheles mosquito. A mosquito belonging to the genus *Anopheles*; many transmit the malaria parasite to people.

Anorexia. Loss of appetite that leads to inability to eat.

Anus. The opening at the end of the alimentary canal through which solid waste passes.

Ascaris lumbricoides. Roundworm, the most common intestinal parasite.

Asphyxiation. Unconsciousness or death caused by lack of oxygen.

Asymptomatic. Exhibiting no symptoms.

Autoinfection. An infection that is caused by germs, viruses, or parasites that persist on or in the body.

Biopsy. Removal and examination, usually microscopic, of tissue from the living body. A biopsy is performed to establish a precise diagnosis.

Blastocystis hominis. Originally classified as a nonpathogenic yeast, blastocystis is now recognized as a protozoan.

Bloated. Swollen or puffed up, especially as with gas.

Bruxism. Continuous and unconscious grinding of teeth.

Caecum. The large pouch that forms the beginning of the large intestine.

Calabar. Refers to a temporary inflammatory reaction, known as calabar swellings, characteristic of Loa loa infection.

Carcinoma. A malignant tumor originally comprised of epithelial cells.

Cestoda. A class including the tapeworms.

Chorioretinitis. Inflammation of the retina and outer membrane of the eye.

Colic. Acute abdominal pain caused by spasm, obstruction, or distention of any of the hollow viscera.

Collagen. A protein comprised of tiny fibers. It forms connective tissues such as tendons, ligaments, bone, and cartilage.

Complement Fixation Test (comp. fix. test). Test that measures those proteins in blood that are activated by infection.

Congenital. Present at birth but not hereditary.

Corneal ulcers. An inflammatory lesion of the structure that covers the lens of the eye.

Crohn's Disease. An inflammatory bowel disease. The cause of this long-term illness is unknown.

Cryptosporidium. A protozoan known to cause diarrhea in both animals and humans.

Cutaneous. Of or pertaining to the skin.

Cutaneous larva migrans. Syndrome caused by dog and cat hookworm larvae and characterized by lesions on the skin at their point of entrance.

Cyst. A capsule that surrounds and protects the larval stage of some parasites.

Cysticerci. Cyst-like organisms.

Cysticercosis. A condition resulting from infection by pork tapeworm and characterized by seizures and brain deterioration.

Cystoscopy. Visual examination of the urinary tract with a special device called a cystoscope.

Dermatitis. Skin inflammation marked by redness, pain, and/or itching.

Disseminated strongyloides. A sometimes fatal condition caused by the nematode *Strongyloides stercoralis*.

Distention. Condition of being expanded due to or as if from internal pressure.

Duodenum. The shortest and widest part of the small intestine.

Dysentery. Infection in the lower intestinal tract that causes pain, fever, and severe diarrhea.

Ectoparasites. Parasites that live on the body (mites and tics).

Edema. Abnormal accumulation of fluid.

Elephantiasis. Enlargement and hardening of cutaneous and subcutaneous tissue, particularly of legs and scrotum; this condition is the result of lymphatic obstruction caused by a nematode.

Encephalitis. Inflammation of the brain.

Endemic. Prevelant in or unique to a particular place or a particular people.

Encyst. Become enclosed in a sac.

Endolimax nana. A type of very small amoeba that may be pathogenic and cause arthritis in people.

Endoparasites. Parasites that live inside the body.

Endothelial cells. Flat cells that line various cavities and vessels.

Entamoeba coli. A type of amoeba similar to E. histolytica; it may cause diarrhea but is not invasive of the colon mucosa.

Entamoeba hartmanni. An amoeba like E. histolytica but smaller.

Entamoeba histolytica. A variety of ameba that is often responsible for causing an infection of the intestines or liver. (*See* amebiasis.)

Eosinophilia. An increase in the number of eosinophils in the blood.

Eosinophils. A type of white blood cell having two rounded projections, eosinophils comprise 1–3 percent of the total white blood cells. Allergies, some infections, and parasites can cause an increase in their numbers.

Epidemiologist. A person who studies epidemics and epidemic diseases.

Etiology. The study of causes or origins of disease.

Feces. Bodily waste excreted from the bowels.

Failure-to-thrive syndrome. Slowed growth in infants resulting from conditions that affect normal body functions, appetite, and activity.

Fibrosis. The overgrowth of fiberlike connective tissue.

Filariae. Microscopic roundworms.

Filariasis. Parasitic disease caused by *Filaria*, a type of worm.

Flocculation. A phenomena relating to a suspension of finely divided particles in which the disperse phase separates in discrete, usually visible, particles rather than in a continuous mass.

Flukes. Leaf-shaped flatworms.

Fluorescent Antibody Test (F.A.T.). Test that reveals antibodies through the use of fluorescent lighting.

Giardiasis. Parasitic disease caused by *Giardia lamblia*, a Protozoa.

Granulomas. Tumorlike masses.

Ground itch. Itchy patches of skin, pimples, and/or blisters resulting from infection by hookworm larvae.

Hematuria. A condition characterized by the presence of blood or red blood cells in the urine.

Hemagglutination. The clumping of red blood cells into groups or masses.

Hemoptysis. Spitting or coughing up of blood from the lungs or bronchial tubes.

Hepatic. Of or pertaining to the liver.

Hepatomegaly. Abnormal enlargement of the liver.

Histiocytes. Large cells in the reticuloendothelial system that have the ability to surround, eat, and digest small living things.

HIV. Human immunodeficiency virus. This virus attacks blood cells, resulting in suppression of the body's immune system and causing AIDS.

Hookworm. Small parasitic worms of the family Ancylostomatidae. With hooked mouths, these nematodes fasten themselves to the intestinal walls of their hosts.

Host. Organism that serves as the home for the parasite.

Hydrocephalus. A condition marked by an abnormal amount of spinal fluid in the head, enlargement of the skull, and compression of the brain.

Hyperglobulinemia. Excess of globulin in the blood.

Ileum. The portion of the small intestine that opens into the large intestine.

Immunoglobulin. Any of five antibodies found in the serum and external bodily secretions. Formed in response to certain foreign bodies (antigens).

Immunosuppressive drugs. Substances that reduce or halt immune response.

Immune response. Manner in which the body's defense system fights invasive bacteria, virus, allergens, and parasites.

Infectious. Having the capacity to cause infection.

Intradermal. Within the layer of the skin that contains the nerve endings, sweat glands, and blood and lymph vessels.

Irritable bowel syndrome. Greatly increased movement of the intestines—both small and large—often associated with stress.

Lactose. Sugar found in milk.

Larvae. The earliest stage of a newly hatched insect, often wormlike.

Leishmaniasis. An infection caused by a protozoan parasite that is transmitted by sand flies. It causes uclers of nose, mouth, throat, and ears.

Lesion. A wound, injury, or circumscribed alteration of tissue caused by disease.

Leukocytosis. A significant increase in the number of white or colorless nucleated blood cells.

Leukopenia. Abnormal decrease in the number of white blood cells.

Lumen. The inner, open space in an organ.

Lymphangitis. An inflammation of one or more of the lymphatic vessels.

Lymphatic. Of or pertaining to the system of nodes and vessels that transport lymph, a bodily fluid that contains white blood cells and some red ones.

Malabsorption. Inadequate or defective absorbing of nutrients from the intestinal tract.

Megacolon. Abnormal and extensive widening of the large intestine.

Megaesophagus. Abnormal widening of the lower parts of the esophagus.

Methylene blue dye. Dye used in a lab test, helps contrast bacteria or parasites so that they are more easily seen.

Monocytes. The largest white blood cells; they are two to four times as large as red blood cells.

Moribund. Approaching death.

Mucosa. A membrane that lines bodily channels that communicate with the air.

Myocarditis. Inflammation of the muscle tissue of the heart.

Nematoda. The phylum name for unsegmented threadlike worms such as the hookworm.

Nephritis. Inflammation of the kidneys.

Night soil. Human excrement used as fertilizer.

Nodule aspirate. Removal of fluids from a nodule by suction.

Ocular larva migrans. Form of visceral larva migrans that infects the eye.

Onchocerciasis. Known as "river blindness," this condition is caused by the filaria *Onchocerca.*

Oocysts. The encysted form of some sporozoan eggs.

Papular. Characterized by small solid skin bumps.

Parenchyma. The tissue that is characteristic of an organ rather than its supporting or connective tissue.

Pathogen. That which causes disease.

Parasite. An animal or plant that grows, feeds, and is sheltered in or on another organism but contributes nothing to the survival of that host organism.

Parasitism. The condition in which an organism obtains its needs from another organism that it is living in or on it.

Perianal. About or around the anus.

Peritoneum. The membrane that covers the wall of the abdomen and is folded over inner organs.

Pernicious anemia. A disorder marked by inadequate production of red blood cells resulting from a nutritional deficit such as lack of iron, folic acid, or vitamin B-12.

Pinworms. *Enterobius vermicularis,* nematode worm that infects the intestines and rectum.

Pleurisy. Inflammation of one or both of the membranous sacs that line the chest cavity and envelope the lungs.

Pneumocystic carinii. Parasite that causes a lung infection (pneumocystosis).

Pneumonitis. Inflammation of the lung.

Polymorphonuclear (P.M.N.). White blood cell that is a granular leukocyte or neutrophil.

Porcine. Of or resembling pigs or swine.

Proglottids. A segment of a tapeworm that contains both the male and female reproductive organs.

Prophylaxis. Prevention or protective treatment.

Prostaglandin. A hormonelike substance found in various human body tissues. Prostaglandins may affect blood pressure, metabolism, and smooth muscle activity.

Protozoa. Single-celled organisms; the most primitive form of animal life.

Pulmonary. Of or pertaining to the lungs.

Roundworms. Of the class Nematoda, roundworms may

be both parasitic or free living with muscles running the length of their bodies.

Schistosomes. Blood flukes.

Schistosomiasis. Infection caused by the *Schistosoma* parasitic worm often found in water contaminated with human waste.

Scolex. Head of a tapeworm that attaches to the intestinal wall.

Scrotum. The external sac of skin that encloses the testes.

Serology. The study of antigen-antibody reactions in a test tube.

Sonogram. From "sono" meaning sound. An image produced by ultrasonography, a sonogram is also called an echogram, sonograph, or ultrasonogram and is a technique in which sound waves are transmitted to hard-to-reach body areas and their echoes are recorded and studied.

Sputum. Material brought up from the lungs and coughed out.

Strabismus. Disorder of the eye muscles in which both eyes cannot be focused on the same point at the same time.

Striated muscle. Voluntary muscles comprised of bundles of parallel fibers.

Strongyloides. A nematode or small roundworm.

Tapeworm. Long parasitic flatworm of the class Cestoda; inhabits the intestines.

Toxocaria canis. Dog roundworms that cause a disease calleed visceral larva migrans in humans, mainly children.

Toxocaria cati. Cat roundworms that cause a disease called visceral larva migrans in humans, mainly children.

Toxoplasma gondii. Intracellular parasite of birds and mammals (particularly cats) that can infect people.

Toxoplasmosis. Disease caused by *Toxoplasma gondii*, marked by tissue alteration in the brain and eye with lesions affecting the lungs, liver, heart, and muscles.

Trematoda. Leaf-shaped flatworms also known as flukes.

Trichomonas vaginalis. A parasitic protozoan that is widespread in humans. It lives in the vagina and sometimes causes inflammation, itching, and burning. It is also found in the male reproductive system.

Trophozoite. A protozoan of the Sporozoa class in the active stage.

Trophs. Short for trophozoite.

Ulceration. Development of a lesion on an internal mucous surface.

Vector. Agent that carries or transmits the infecting pathogen.

Vermifuge. A substance that expels or destroys intestinal worms.

Visceral larva migrans. A condition resulting from invasion of human viscera by nematode larva.

Volvulus. Intestinal obstruction caused by abnormal twisting.

Winterbottom's sign. A lymph condition at the base of the skull.

Notes

Chapter 1
What You Don't Know Can
Hurt You

1. Centers for Disease Control, *Malaria Surveillance Annual Summary 1989*, issued November 1990.
2. L. Parrish, "The Protozoal Syndrome," *Townsend Letter for Doctors* (December 1990) 832.
3. "Technology, Funds Promise New Era in Parasitology," *Journal of the American Medical Association* 252 (December 14, 1984): 3081.
4. Terry Kay Rockefeller, *Conquest of the Parasites*, produced by Paula Apsell, PBS, January 29, 1985, transcript, p. 8.
5. Centers for Disease Control, *Malaria Surveillance Annual Summary 1989*.
6. Jane Brody, "Test Unmasks a Parasitic Disease," *New York Times*, 26 October 1989, sec. B, p. 12.
7. L. Galland, et al., "Giardia lambla Infection as a Cause of Chronic Fatigue," *Journal of Nutritional Medicine* 1 (1990): 27–31.
8. S. Rochlitz, *Allergies and Candida* (New York: Human Ecology Balancing Sciences, Inc., 1991) 100.
9. P.W. Moser, "Danger in Diaperland," *In Health*, September–October 1991, 78.
10. *Ibid.*
11. William Blair, "Disease Is Cited in Veterans' Suit," *New York Times*, 24 July 1985, Sec. 2, p. 2.
12. Juan Walte, "Gulf War Parasite Halts Troop Blood Drive,"

USA Today, 13 November 1991, sec. A, p. 1.

13. M. Rosenbaum and M. Susser, *Solving the Puzzle of Chronic Fatigue Syndrome* (Tacoma, WA: Life Sciences Press, 1992), 51.

14. International Medical News Service, "Animal-Transmitted Diseases Often Unsuspected, Unrecognized," *Pediatric News* 11 (September 1977): 9.

15. C. Lane, et al., A Letter to the Editor, "If Your Uneaten Food Moves, Take it to a Doctor," *Journal of the American Medical Association* 260 (July 15, 1988): 340.

16. J. McKerrow, et al., "Anisakiasis: Revenge of the Sushi Parasite," *New England Journal of Medicine* 319 (November 3, 1988): 1228.

17. W. Petri and J. Ravdin, "Treatment of Homosexual Men Infected With Entamoeba histolytica," *New England Journal of Medicine* 315 (August 7, 1986): 393.

Chapter 3
Guide to Parasites

1. Alison Cook, "Unwelcome Guest, Reluctant Host," *Texas Monthly*, May 1985, 166–168.

2. Robert McCabe, and Jack Remington, "Toxoplasmosis: The Time Has Come," *New England Journal of Medicine* 318 (February 1988):313–315.

Chapter 4
The Water and Food Connection

1. Voge and John Markell, *Medical Parasitology, 6th Edition*, (Philadelphia: W.B. Saunders Co., 1986), 58.

2. Moser, "Danger In Diaperland," 77–80.

3. J.H. Thompson, "Times, Manners, and the STD List: An Essay," *Laboratory Management*, July 1984, 16.

4. Jeanette K. Stehr-Green and Theodore Bailey, et al., "Acanthamoeba Keratitis in Soft Contact Lens Wearers," *Journal of the American Medical Association* 258 (July 3, 1987):57–60.

5. R. Gregory, et al., "Acute Schistosomiasis Among Americans Rafting in the Omo River, Ethiopia," *Journal of the American Medical Association* 251 (January 27, 1984):508–510.

6. Wilbur Cross and Thorleif Hellbom, "Long Journey to Nowhere," *Wide World*, February 1963, 85–134.

7. M. Wittner, "Eustrongylides— A Parasitic Infection Acquired by Eating Sushi," *New England Journal of Medicine* 320 (April 27, 1989):1124–1126.

8. Lane, "If Your Uneaten Food Moves, Take it to a Doctor," 340–341.

9. Shirley Mandel, "Nutrition for Better Health," *Jewish Press*, 8 April 1988, sec. M, p. 34–35.

Chapter 5
Man's Best Friend

1. "Be My Hospital Buddy," *Medical Tribune*, March 25, 1987.
2. D. Elliot, et al., "Pet Associated Illness," *New England Journal of Medicine* 313 (October 17, 1985):985–995.
3. International Medical News Service, "Animal-Transmitted Diseases Often Unsuspected, Unrecognized," 9.
4. S. Bechtel, "What You Can and Cannot Catch From A Pet," *Prevention*, April 1984, 71.
5. Marjorie V. Baldwin, "We Love Animals, But . . ." *Wildwood Echoes*, Spring 1981, 3.
6. S. Teutsch, et al., "Epidemic Toxoplasmosis Associated with Infected Cats," *New England Journal of Medicine*, 300 (March 29, 1979):695–699.
7. R. McCabe and J.S. Remington, "Toxoplasmosis: The Time Has Come," *New England Journal of Medicine* 318 (February 4, 1988):313–315.

Chapter 7
Diagnosis

1. S. Baron, editor, *Medical Microbiology, 3rd Edition* (New York: Churchill Livingstone, 1991), 1041.
2. *Ibid.*
3. Parrish, "The Protozoal Syndrome," 832–835.
4. Baron, 989.
5. L. Dowell, "Stool Examinations—A Procedure to Increase Their Value," *Official Journal of A.M.T.* (January–February 1961).
6. Brody, "Test Unmasks a Parasitic Disease," p. 12.
7. M.S. Wolfe, "Diseases of Travelers," *CIBA Clinical Symposia* 36 (November 2, 1984): 28.

Chapter 8
Treatment

1. D. Mirelman, et al., "Inhibition of Growth of Entamoeba histoyltica by Allicin, the Active Principle of Garlic Extract," *Journal of Infectious Diseases* 156(1):243–244, 1987.
2. "How to Fight Off Parasites and Pathogens—Safely," *Stool Scene*, Great Smokies Diagnostic Laboratory (January–March 1987): 3.
3. D.L. Taren, and D.W.T. Crompton, "Nutritional Interactions During Parasitism," *Clinical Nutrition* (November–December 1989): 227–238.
4. D. Mahalanabis, K.N. Jalan, T.K. Maitra, S.K. Agarwal, "Vitamin A Absorption in Ascariasis," *American Journal of Clinical Nutrition* 29 (1976): 372–375.
5. D. Mahalanabis, T.W. Simpson, M.L. Chakroborty, et al., "Malabsorption of Water Mis-

cible Vitamin A in Children With Giardiasis and Ascariasis," *American Journal of Clinical Nutrition* 321 (1979): 313–318.

6. E.P. Veriyam and J.G. Banwell, "Hookworm Disease: Nutritional Implications," Reviews of Infectious Diseases, (1982): 830–835.

7. Taren and Crompton, "Nutritional Interactions During Parasitism," 227–238.

8. *Ibid.*

9. C. Krakower, W.A. Hoffman, and J.H. Axtmayer, "The Fate of Schistosomes (S.mansoni) in Experimental Infections of Normal and Vitamin A Deficient White Rats," *Puerto Rico Journal of Public Health Tropical Medicine* 16 (1940): 269–345.

10. R.E. Gingrich, and C.C. Barett, "Effect of Dietary Vitamin A on the Innate Resistance of Cattle to Infestation by Larvae of *Hypoderma lineatum* (Deptera:Oestride)," *Journal of Medical Entomology* 12 (1975): 13–15.

11. L.D. Stephenson, et al., "Relationships Between *Ascaris* Infection and Growth of Malnourished Pre-school Children in Kenya," *American Journal of Clinical Nutrition* 33 (1980):1165–1172.

12. G. Leitch, et al., "Dietary Fiber and Giardiasis," *American Journal of Tropical Medicine and Hygiene* 41(5):512–520, 1989.

13. "Giardiasis: An Update," *Infectious Disease Practice* 1 (1978): 1–5.

14. Taren and Crompton, "Nutritional Interactions During Parasitism," 227–238.

15. *Ibid.*

16. "Keep the Bile Away From Giardia!" *Stool Scene,* Great Smokies Diagnostic Laboratory (Winter 1990): 3.

17. "Drugs for Parasitic Infections," *The Medical Letter on Drugs and Therapeutics* (March 6, 1992): 1.

18. Parrish, "The Protozoan Syndrome," 832–835.

19. T. Mitsuoka, H. Hidaka, and T. Eida, "Effect of Fructo-Oligosaccharides on Intestinal Microflora," *Die Nahrung,* 31 (1987): 427–436.

Chapter 10

Closing Comments

1. Baron, 966

2. *Ibid.,* 1126.

Suggested Reading List

De Schepper, Luc. *Full of Life*. Los Angeles: Tale Weaver Publishing, 1991.

*Di Fabio, Anthony. *Rheumatoid Diseases Cured At Last*. Franklin, Tennessee: The Rheumatoid Disease Foundation, 1982.

Gittleman Ann Louise. *Beyond Pritikin*. New York: Bantam Books, 1988.

**Litter, Leo. "Pinworms—A Ten Year Study." *Archives of Pediatrics 78 (November 1961): 440–455*.

Rosenbaum, Michael and Susser, Murray. *Solving the Puzzle of Chronic Fatigue Syndrome*. Tacoma, Washington: Life Sciences Press, 1992.

*Wynburn-Mason, Roger. *The Causation of Rheumatoid Disease and Many Human Cancers: A New Concept in Medicine*. Tokyo: Iji Publishing Company, 1978.

*Write to the Rheumatoid Disease Foundation, Route 4, Box 137, Franklin, Tennessee 37064 to obtain copies.

**For reprints, write to Dr. Leo Litter, 16 High Ridge Road, West Hartford, Connecticut 06117.

Appendix

This section is a reprint of the March 6, 1992, issue of "The Medical Letter." It contains information your physician may find helpful in treating parasitic infections. There is a listing of antiparasitic drugs as well as specific treatment dosages for particular infections.

DRUGS FOR PARASITIC INFECTIONS

Parasitic infections are now found throughout the world. With increasing travel, use of immunosuppressive drugs, and the spread of AIDS, physicians anywhere may see infections caused by previously unfamiliar parasites. The table that begins on the next page lists first-choice and alternative drugs for most parasitic infections. In every case, the need for treatment must be weighed against the toxicity of the drug. A decision to withhold therapy may often be correct, particularly when the drugs can cause severe adverse effects. When the first-choice drug is initially ineffective and the alternative is more hazardous, it may be prudent to try a second course of treatment with the first drug before using the alternative. Adverse effects of some antiparasitic drugs are also listed, beginning on page 181.

PARTIAL LIST OF ANTIPARASITIC DRUGS

*albendazole—*Zentel* (SmithKline Beecham)
**benznidazole—*Rochagan* (Roche, Brazil)
***bithionol—Bitin (Tanabe, Japan)
chloroquine—*Aralen* (Sanofi Winthrop), others
crotamiton—*Eurax* (Westwood-Squibb)
***dehydroemetine—(Hoffmann-LaRoche, Switzerland)
*diethylcarbamazine—*Hetrazan* (Lederle), others
***diloxanide furoate—*Furamide* (Boots, England)
*eflornithine (difluoromethylornithine, DFMO)—*Ornidyl* (Merrell Dow)
**flubendazole—(Janssen)
furazolidone—*Furoxone* (Roberts)
**halofantrine—*Halfan* (SmithKline Beecham)
hydroxychloroquine—*Plaquenil* (Sanofi Winthrop)
iodoquinol (diiodohydroxyquin)—*Yodoxin* (Glenwood), others
***ivermectin—*Mectizan* (Merck)
lindane (gamma benzene hexachloride)—*Kwell* (Reed & Carnrick), others
malathion—*Ovide* (GenDerm)
mebendazole—*Vermox* (Janssen)
mefloquine—*Lariam* (Roche)
**meglumine antimoniate—*Glucantime* (Rhône-Poulenc Rorer, France)
***melarsoprol—*Arsobal* (Rhône-Poulenc Rorer, France)
metronidazole—*Flagyl* (Searle), others
niclosamide—*Niclocide* (Miles)
***nifurtimox—*Lampit* (Bayer, Germany)

**ornidazole—*Tiberal* (Hoffmann-LaRoche, Switzerland)
oxamniquine—*Vansil* (Pfizer)
paromomycin—*Humatin* (Parke-Davis)
pentamidine isethionate—*Pentam 300* (Fujisawa), *NebuPent* (Fujisawa)
permethrin—*Nix* (Burroughs Wellcome), *Elimite* (Herbert)
praziquantel—*Biltricide* (Miles)
primaquine phosphate—(Sanofi Winthrop)
**proguanil—*Paludrine* (Ayerst, Canada, ICI, England)
pyrantel pamoate—*Antiminth* (Pfizer)
pyrethrins and piperonyl butoxide—*RID* (Pfizer), others
pyrimethamine—*Daraprim* (Burroughs Wellcome)
pyrimethamine-sulfadoxine—*Fansidar* (Roche)
quinacrine—*Atabrine* (Sanofi Winthrop)
quinidine gluconate—many manufacturers
**quinine dihydrochloride
quinine sulfate—many manufacturers
*spiramycin—*Rovamycine* (Rhône-Poulenc Rorer)
***stibogluconate sodium (antimony sodium gluconate)—*Pentostam* (Burroughs Wellcome, England)
***suramin—*Germanin* (Bayer, Germany)
thiabendazole—*Mintezol* (Merck)
**tinidazole—*Fasigyn* (Pfizer)
**triclabendazole (Ciba-Geigy, France)
****trimetrexate—(US Bioscience)
**tryparsamide

*Available in the USA only from the manufacturer
**Not available in the USA
***Available from the CDC Drug Service, Centers for Disease Control, Atlanta, Georgia 30333; 404–639–3670 (evenings, weekends, or holidays: 404–639–2888)
****Available from the National Institute of Allergy and Infectious Diseases, 1–800–537–9978

DRUGS FOR TREATMENT OF PARASITIC INFECTIONS

Infection	Drug	Adult Dosage*	Pediatric Dosage*
AMEBIASIS (*Entamoeba histolytica*)			
asymptomatic			
Drug of choice:	Iodoquinol[1]	650 mg tid x 20d	30–40 mg/kg/d in 3 doses x 20d
	OR		
	Paromomycin	25–30 mg/kg/d in 3 doses x 7d	25–30 mg/kg/d in 3 doses x 7d
Alternative:	Diloxànide furoate[2]	500 mg tid x 10d	20 mg/kg/d in 3 doses x 10d
mild to moderate intestinal disease			
Drugs of choice:	Metronidazole[3]	750 mg tid x 10d	35–50 mg/kg/d in 3 doses x 10d
	OR		
	Tinidazole[4] **followed by**	2 grams/d x 3d	50 mg/kg (max. 2 grams) qd x 3d
	iodoquinol[1]	650 mg tid x 20d	30–40 mg/kg/d in 3 doses x 20d
	OR		
	paromomycin	25–30 mg/kg/d in 3 doses x 7d	25–30 mg/kg/d in 3 doses x 7d
severe intestinal disease			
Drugs of choice:	Metronidazole[3]	750 mg tid x 10d	35–50 mg/kg/d in 3 doses x 10d
	OR		
	Tinidazole[4] **followed by**	600 mg bid x 5d	50 mg/kg (max. 2 grams) qd x 3d
	iodoquinol[1]	650 mg tid x 20d	30–40 mg/kg/d in 3 doses x 20d
	OR		
	paromomycin	25–30 mg/kg/d in 3 doses x 7d	25–30 mg/kg/d in 3 doses x 7d
Alternatives:	Dehydroemetine[2,5]	1 to 1.5 mg/kg/d (max. 90 mg/d) IM of up to 5d	1 to 1.5 mg/kg/d (max. 90 mg/d) IM in 2 doses for up to 5d
	followed by		
	iodoquinol[1]	650 mg tid x 20d	30–40 mg/kg/d in 3 doses x 20d
hepatic abscess			
Drugs of choice:	Metronidazole[3]	750 mg tid x 10d	35–50 mg/kg/d in 3 doses x 10d
	OR		
	Tinidazole[4] **followed by**	800 mg tid x 5d	60 mg/kg (max. 2 grams) qd x 3d
	iodoquinol[1]	650 mg tid x 20d	30–40 mg/kg/d in 3 doses x 20d
Alternatives:	Dehydroemetine[2,5]	1 to 1.5 mg/kg/d (max. 90 mg/d) IM for up to 5d	1 to 1.5 mg/kg/d (max. 90 mg/d) IM in 2 doses for up to 5d

Infection	Drug	Adult Dosage*	Pediatric Dosage*

AMEBIASIS (*Entamoeba histolytica*), treatment with hepatic abscess *(continued)*

Alternatives:	**followed by** chloroquine phosphate	600 mg base (1 gram)/d x 2d, then 300 mg base (500 mg)/d x 2–3 wks	10 mg base/kg (max. 300 mg base)/d x 2–3 wks
	plus iodoquinol[1]	650 mg tid x 20d	30–40 mg/kg/d in 3 doses x 20d

AMEBIC MENINGOENCEPHALITIS, PRIMARY

Naegleria

Drug of choice:	Amphotericin B[6,7]	1 mg/kg/d IV, uncertain duration	1 mg/kg/d IV, uncertain duration

Acanthamoeba

Drug of choice:	see footnote 8		

Ancylostoma duodenale, See HOOKWORM

ANGIOSTRONGYLIASIS

Angiostrongylus cantonensis

Drug of choice:	Mebendazole[7,9,10]	100 mg bid x 5d	100 mg bid x 5d

Angiostrongylus costaricensis

Drug of choice:	Thiabendazole[7,9]	75 mg/kg/d in 3 doses x 3d[11] (max. 3 grams/d)	75 mg/kg/d in 3 doses x 3d[11] (max 3 grams/d)

ANISAKIASIS (*Anisakis*)

Treatment of choice:	Surgical or endoscopic removal		

ASCARIASIS (*Ascaris lumbricoides*, roundworm)

Drug of choice:	Mebendazole	100 mg bid x 3d	100 mg bid x 3d
	OR		
	Pyrantel pamoate	11 mg/kg once (max. 1 gram)	11 mg/kg once (max. 1 gram)
	OR		
	Albendazole	400 mg once	400 mg once

Infection	Drug	Adult Dosage*	Pediatric Dosage*
BABESIOSIS (*Babesia*)			
Drugs of choice:[12]	Clindamycin[7]	1.2 grams bid parenteral or 600 mg tid oral x 7d	20–40 mg/kg/d in 3 doses x 7d
	plus quinine	650 mg tid oral x 7d	25 mg/kg/d in 3 doses x 7d
BALANTIDIASIS (*Balantidium coli*)			
Drug of choice:	Tetracycline[7]	500 mg qid x 10d	40 mg/kg/d in 4 doses x 10d (max. 2 grams/d)[13]
Alternatives:	Iodoquinol[1,7]	650 mg tid x 20d	40 mg/kg/d in 3 doses x 20d
	Metronidazole[3,7]	750 mg tid x 5d	35–50 mg/kg/d in 3 doses x 5d
BAYLISASCARIASIS (*Baylisascaris procyonis*)			
Drug of choice:	See footnote 14		
BLASTOCYSTIS hominis infection			
Drug of choice:	See footnote 15		
CAPILLARIASIS (*Capillaria philippinensis*)			
Drug of choice:	Mebendazole[7]	200 mg bid x 20d	200 mg bid x 20d
Alternatives:	Albendazole	200 mg bid x 10d	200 mg bid x 10d
	Thiabendazole[7]	25 mg/kg/d in 2 doses x 30d	25 mg/kg/d in 2 doses x 30d
Chagas' disease, *See* TRYPANOSOMIASIS			
***Clonorchis sinensis*, *See* FLUKE infection**			
CRYPTOSPORIDIOSIS (*Cryptosporidium*)			
Drug of choice:	See footnote 16		
CUTANEOUS LARVA MIGRANS (creeping eruption)			
Drug of choice:[17]	Thiabendazole	Topically and/or 50 mg/kg/d in 2 doses (max. 3 grams/d) x 2–5d[11]	Topically and/or 50 mg/kg/d in 2 doses (max .3 grams/d) x 2–5d[11]
Cysticercosis, *See* TAPEWORM infection			

Infection	Drug	Adult Dosage*	Pediatric Dosage*
DIENTAMOEBA *fragilis* infection			
Drug of choice:	Iodoquinol[1]	650 mg tid x 20d	40 mg/kg/d in 3 doses x 20d
	OR		
	Paromomycin	25–30 mg/kg/d in 3 doses x 7d	25–30 mg/kg/d in 3 doses x 7d
	OR		
	Tetracycline[7]	500 mg qid x 10d	40 mg/kg/d in 4 doses x 10d (max. 2 grams/d)[13]

Diphyllobothrium latum, *See* TAPEWORM infection

DRACUNCULUS *medinensis* (guinea worm) infection			
Drug of choice:	Metronidazole[3,7,18]	250 mg tid x 10d	25 mg/kg/d (max. 750 mg/d) in 3 doses x 10d
Alternative:	Thiabendazole[7,18]	50–75 mg/kg/d in 2 doses x 3d[11]	50–75 mg/kg/d in 2 doses x 3d[11]

Echinococcus, *See* TAPEWORM infection

Entamoeba histolytica, *See* AMEBIASIS

ENTAMOEBA *polecki* infection			
Drug of choice:	Metronidazole[3,7]	750 mg tid x 10d	35–50 mg/kg/d in 3 doses x 10d

ENTEROBIUS *vermicularis* (pinworm) infection			
Drug of choice:	Pyrantel pamoate	11 mg/kg once (max. 1 gram); repeat after 2 weeks	11 mg/kg once (max. 1 gram); repeat after 2 weeks
	OR		
	Mebendazole	A single dose of 100 mg; repeat after 2 weeks	A single dose of 100 mg; repeat after 2 weeks
	OR		
	Albendazole	400 mg once; repeat in 2 weeks	400 mg once; repeat in 2 weeks

Fasciola hepatica, *See* FLUKE infection

FILARIASIS

Wuchereria bancrofti, Brugia malayi

Drug of choice:[19]   Diethylcarbamazine[20]   Day 1: 50 mg, oral, p.c.   Day 1: 1 mg/kg, oral, p.c.

Infection	Drug	Adult Dosage*	Pediatric Dosage*
FILARIASIS, treatment of *Wuchereria bancrofti, Brugia malayi* (continued)			
		Day 2: 50 mg tid	Day 2: 1 mg/kg/tid
		Day 3: 100 mg tid	Day 3: 1–2 mg/kg tid
		Days 4 through 21: 6 mg/kg/d in 3 doses[21]	Days 4 through 21: 6 mg/kg/d in 3 doses[21]
Loa loa			
Drug of choice:	Diethylcarba-mazine[20]	Day 1: 50 mg, oral, p.c.	Day 1: 1 mg/kg, oral, p.c.
		Day 2: 50 mg tid	Day 2: 1 mg/kg tid
		Day 3: 100 mg tid	Day 3: 1–2 mg/kg tid
		Days 4 through 21: 9 mg/kg/d in 3 doses[21]	Days 4 through 21: 9 mg/kg/d in 3 doses[21]
Mansonella ozzardi			
Drug of choice:	See footnote 19		
Mansonella perstans			
Drug of choice:[22]	Mebendazole[7]	100 mg bid x 30d	
Tropical Pulmonary Eosinophilia (TPE)			
Drug of choice:	Diethylcarbamazine	6 mg/kg/d in 3 doses x 21d	6 mg/kg/d in 3 doses x 21d
Onchocerca volvulus			
Drug of choice:	Ivermectin[2]	150 µg/kg oral once, repeated every 6 to 12 months	150 µg/kg oral once, repeated every 6 to 12 months
FLUKE, hermaphroditic, infection			
Clonorchis sinensis (Chinese liver fluke)			
Drug of choice:	Praziquantel	75 mg/kg/d in 3 doses	75 mg/kg/d in 3 doses
Fasciola hepatica (sheep liver fluke)			
Drug of choice:[23]	Bithionol[2]	30–50 mg/kg on alternate days x 10–15 doses	30–50 mg/kg on alternate days x 10–15 doses

Infection	Drug	Adult Dosage*	Pediatric Dosage*

FLUKE, hermaphroditic, infection *(continued)*

Fasciolopsis buski (intestinal fluke)

Drug of choice:	Praziquantel[7]	75 mg/kg/d in 3 doses x 1d	75 mg/kg/d in 3 doses x 1d
	OR		
	Niclosamide[7]	a single dose of 4 tablets (2 g), chewed thoroughly	11–34 kg: 2 tablets (1 g) > 34 kg: 3 tablets (1.5 g)

Heterophyes heterophyes (intestinal fluke)

Drug of choice	Praziquantel[7]	75 mg/kg/d in 3 doses x 1d	75 mg/kg/d in 3 doses x 1d

Metagonimus yokogawai (intestinal fluke)

Drug of choice:	Praziquantel[7]	75 mg/kg/d in 3 doses x 1d	75 mg/kg/d in 3 doses x 1d

Nanophyetus salmincola

Drug of choice:	Praziquantel[7]	60 mg/kg/d in 3 doses x 1d	60 mg/kg/d in 3 doses x 1d

Opisthorchis viverrini (liver fluke)

Drug of choice:	Praziquantel	75 mg/kg/d in 3 doses x 1d	75 mg/kg/d in 3 doses x 1d

Paragonimus westermani (lung fluke)

Drug of choice:	Praziquantel[7]	75 mg/kg/d in 3 doses x 2d	75 mg/kg/d in 3 doses x 2d
Alternative	Bithionol[2]	30–50 mg/kg on alternate days x 10–15 doses	30–50 mg/kg on alternate days x 10–15 doses

GIARDIASIS *(Giardia intestinalis*, formerly *G. lamblia)*

Drug of choice:	Quinacrine HCl	100 mg tid p.c. x 5d	6 mg/kg/d in 3 doses p.c. x 5d (max. 300 mg/d)
Alternatives:	Metronidazole[3,7]	250 mg tid x 5d	15 mg/kg/d in 3 doses x 5d
	Tinidazole[4]	2 grams once	50 mg/kg once (max. 2 grams)
	Furazolidone	100 mg qid x 7–10d	
	Paromomycin[24]	25–30 mg/kg/d in 3 doses x 7d	6 mg/kg/d in 4 doses x 7–10d

Infection	Drug	Adult Dosage*	Pediatric Dosage*
GNATHOSTOMIASIS (*Gnathostoma spinigerum*)			
Treatment of choice:	Surgical removal		
	OR		
	Mebendazole[7]	200 mg q3h x 6d	

Infection	Drug	Adult Dosage*	Pediatric Dosage*
HOOKWORM infection (*Ancylostoma duodenale, Necator americanus*)			
Drug of choice:	Mebendazole	100 mg bid x 3d	100 mg bid x 3d
	OR		
	Pyrantel pamoate[7]	11 mg/kg (max. 1 gram) x 3d	11 mg/kg (max. 1 gram) x 3d
	OR		
	Albendazole	400 mg once	400 mg once

Hydatid cyst, *See* TAPEWORM infection

Hymenolepis nana, *See* TAPEWORM infection

Infection	Drug	Adult Dosage*	Pediatric Dosage*
ISOSPORIASIS (*Isospora belli*)			
Drug of choice:	Trimethoprim-sulfamethoxazole[7,25]	160 mg TMP, 800 mg SMX qid x 10d, then bid x 3 wks	

Infection	Drug	Adult Dosage*	Pediatric Dosage*
LEISHMANIASIS (*L. mexicana, L. tropica, L. major, L. braziliensis, L. donovani* [Kala-azar])			
Drug of choice:[26]	Stibogluconate sodium[2]	20 mg Sb/kg/d IV or IM x 20–28d[27]	20 mg Sb/kg/d IV or IM x 20–28d[27]
	OR		
	Meglumine antimoniate	20 mg Sb/kg/d x 20–28d[27]	20 mg Sb/kg/d x 20–28d[27]
Alternatives:[28]	Amphotericin B[7]	0.25 to 1 mg/kg by slow infusion daily or every 2d for up to 8 wks	0.25 to 1 mg/kg by slow infusion daily or every 2d for up to 8 wks
	Pentamidine isethionate[7]	2–4 mg/kg/d IM for up to 15 doses[27]	2–4 mg/kg/d IM for up to 15 doses[27]
	Topical treatment[29]		

Infection	Drug	Adult Dosage*	Pediatric Dosage*
LICE infestation (*Pediculus humanus, capitis, Phthirus pubis*)[30]			
Drug of choice:	1% Permethrin[31]	Topically	Topically
	OR		
	0.5% Malathion	Topically	Topically
Alternatives:	Pyrethrins with piperonyl butoxide	Topically[32]	Topically[32]
	Lindane	Topically[32]	Topically[32]

Loa loa, *See* FILARIASIS

Infection	Drug	Adult Dosage*	Pediatric Dosage*

MALARIA, Treatment of (*Plasmodium falciparum, P. ovale, P. vivax,* and *P. malariae*)

All *Plasmodium* except Chloroquine-Resistant *P. falciparum*

ORAL

Drug of choice:	Chloroquine phosphate[33,34]	600 mg base (1 gram), then 300 mg base (500 mg) 6 hrs later, then 300 mg base (500 mg) at 24 and 48 hrs	10 mg base/kg (max. 600 mg base), then 5 mg base/kg 6 hrs later, then 5 mg base/kg at 24 and 48 hrs

PARENTERAL

Drug of choice:[35]	Quinidine gluconate[7,36]	10 mg/kg loading dose (max. 600 mg) in normal saline slowly over 1 hr, followed by continuous infusion of 0.02 mg/kg/min for 3 days maximum	Same as adult dose
	OR		
	Quinine dihydrochloride[37]	20 mg salt/kg loading dose in 10 ml/kg 5% dextrose over 4 hrs, followed by 10 mg salt/kg over 2–4 hrs q8h (max. 1800 mg/d) until oral therapy can be started	Same as adult dose

Chloroquine-resistant *P. falciparum*[38]

ORAL

Drugs of choice:[39]	Quinine sulfate[40,41] **plus**	650 mg tid x 3d	25 mg/kg/d in 3 doses x 3d
	pyrimethamine-sulfadoxine[42]	3 tablets at once on last day of quinine	< 1 yr: ¼ tablet 1–3 yrs: ½ tablet 4–8 yrs: 1 tablet 9–14 yrs: 2 tablets
	OR		
	plus tetracycline[7,13]	250 mg qid x 7d	20 mg/kg/d in 4 doses x 7d[13]
	OR		
	plus clindamycin[7]	900 mg tid x 3d	20–40 mg/kg/d in 3 doses x 3d
Alternatives:	Mefloquine[43,44]	1250 mg once[45]	25 mg/kg once[46] (< 45 kg)
	Halofantrine[47]	500 mg q6h x 3 doses	8 mg/kg q6h x 3 doses (< 40 kg)

Infection	Drug	Adult Dosage*	Pediatric Dosage*

MALARIA , Treatment of Chloroquine-resistant *P. Falciparum (continued)*

PARENTERAL

Drug of choice:	Quinidine gluco-nate[7,36]	same as above	same as above
	OR		
	Quinine dihydro-chloride[37]	same as above	same as above

Prevention of relapses: *P. vivax and P. ovale* only

Drug of choice:	Primaquine phosphate[48]	15 mg base (26.3 mg)/d x 14 d or 45 mg base (79 mg)/wk x 8 wks	0.3 mg base/kg/d x 14d

MALARIA, Prevention of[49]

Chloroquine-sensitive areas

Drug of choice:	Chloroquine phos-phate[50]	300 mg base (500 mg salt) orally, once/week beginning 1 week before and continuing for 4 weeks after last exposure	5 mg/kg base (8.3 mg/kg salt) once/week, up to adult dose of 300 mg base

Chloroquine-resistant areas[38]

Drug of choice:[51]	Mefloquine[44,50,52]	250 mg oral once/week[53]	15–19 kg: ¼ tablet 20–30 kg: ½ tablet 31–45 kg: ¾ tablet > 45 kg: 1 tablet
	OR		
	Doxycycline[7,50,54]	100 mg daily	> 8 years of age: 2 mg/kg/d orally, up to 100 mg/day
	OR		
	Chloroquine phosphate[50]	as above	as above
	plus		
	pyrimethamine-sulfadoxine[42] for presumptive treat-ment[55]	Carry a single dose (3 tablets) for self-treatment of febrile illness when medi-cal care is not im-mediately available	< 1 yr: ¼ tablet 1–3 yrs: ½ tablet 4–8 yrs: 1 tablet 9–14 yrs: 2 tablets
	OR plus		
	proguanil[56] (in Africa south of the Sahara)	200 mg daily during exposure and for 4 weeks afterwards	< 2 yrs: 50 mg daily 2–6 yrs: 100 mg daily 7–10 yrs: 150 mg daily 10 yrs: 200 mg daily

Infection	Drug	Adult Dosage*	Pediatric Dosage*
MICROSPORIDIOSIS			
Enterocytozoon bieneusi			
Drug of choice:	none[57]		
Encephalitozoon hellem			
Drug of choice:	none[58]		
Mites, *See* SCABIES			
MONILIFORMIS moniliformis infection			
Drug of choice:	Pyrantel pamoate[7]	11 mg/kg once, repeat twice, 2 wks apart	11 mg/kg once, repeat twice, 2 wks apart
Naegleria species, *See* AMEBIC MENINGOENCEPHALITIS, PRIMARY			
Necator americanus, *See* HOOKWORM infection			
Onchocerca volvulus, *See* FILARIASIS			
Opisthorchis viverrini, *See* FLUKE infection			
Paragonimus westermani, *See* FLUKE infection			
Pediculus capitis, humanus, Phthirus pubis, see LICE			
Pinworm, *See* ENTEROBIUS			
PNEUMOCYSTIS carinii pneumonia[59]			
Drug of choice:	Trimethoprim-sulfamethoxazole	TMP 15–20 mg/kg/d, SMX 75–100 mg/kg/d, oral or IV in 3 or 4 doses x 14–21d	Same as adult dose
	OR		
	Pentamidine	3–4 mg/kg IV qd x 14–21 days	Same as adult dose
Alternatives:	Trimethoprim[7]	5 mg/kg PO q6h x 21 days	
	plus dapsone[7,60]	100 mg PO qd x 21 days	
	Primaquine[7,48]	15 mg base PO qd x 21 days	
	plus clindamycin[7]	600 mg IV q6h x 21 days, or 300–450 mg PO q6h x 21 days	

Infection	Drug	Adult Dosage*	Pediatric Dosage*

PNEUMOCYSTIS *carinii* pneumonia[59] *(continued)*

| | Trimetrexate | 45 mg/m^2 IV qd x 21 days | |
| | **plus** folinic acid | 20 mg/m^2 PO or IV q6h x 21 days | |

Primary and secondary prophylaxis

Drug of choice:	Trimethoprim-sulfamethoxazole	1 DS[61] tab PO qd, bid, or 3x/week	
Alternatives:	Dapsone[7,60]	25–50 mg PO qd, or 100 mg PO 2x week	
	Aerosol pentamidine	300 mg inhaled monthly via *Respirgard II* nebulizer	

Roundworm, *See* ASCARIASIS

SCABIES *(Sarcoptes scabiei)*

Drug of Choice:	5% Permethrin	Topically	Topically
	Lindane[32]	Topically	Topically
	10% Crotamiton	Topically	Topically

SCHISTOSOMIASIS *(Bilharziasis)*

S. haematobium

| Drug of choice: | Praziquantel | 40 mg/kg/d in 2 doses x 1d | 40 mg/kg/d in 2 doses x 1d |

S. japonicum

| Drug of choice: | Praziquantel | 60 mg/kg/d in 3 doses x 1d | 60 mg/kg/d in 3 doses x 1d |

S. mansoni

| Drug of choice: | Praziquantel | 40 mg/kg/d in 2 doses x 1d | 40 mg/kg/d in 2 doses x 1d |
| Alternative: | Oxamniquine[62] | 15 mg/kg once[63] | 20 mg/kg/d in 2 doses x 1d[63] |

S. mekongi

| Drug of choice: | Praziquantel | 60 mg/kg/d in 3 doses x 1d | 60 mg/kg/d in 3 doses x 1d |

Sleeping sickness, *See* TRYPANOSOMIASIS

Infection	Drug	Adult Dosage*	Pediatric Dosage*
STRONGYLOIDIASIS (*Strongyloides stercoralis*)			
Drug of choice:[64]	Thiabendazole	50 mg/kg/d in 2 doses (max. 3 grams/d) x 2d[11,65]	50 mg/kg/d in 2 doses (max. 3 grams/d) x 2d[11,65]
	OR		
	Ivermectin[2]	200 mg/kg/d x 1A2d	
	OR		
	Albendazole	400 mg qd x 3d	400 mg qd x 3d

TAPEWORM infection—Adult (intestinal stage)

Diphyllobothrium latum (fish), Taenia saginata (beef), Taenia solium (pork), Dipylidium caninum (dog)

Drug of choice:	Praziquantel[7]	10–20 mg/kg once	10–20 mg/kg once
	OR		
	Niclosamide	A single dose of 4 tablets (2 grams), chewed thoroughly	11–34 kg: a single dose of 2 tablets (1 gram); >34 kg: a single dose of 3 tablets (1.5 grams)

Hymenolepis nana (dwarf tapeworm)

Drug of choice:	Praziquantel[7]	25 mg/kg once	25 mg/kg once
Alternative:	Niclosamide	A single daily dose of 4 tablets (2 g), chewed thoroughly, then 2 tablets daily x 6d	11–34 kg: a single dose of 2 tablets (1 g) x 1d, then 1 tablet (0.5 grams)/d x 6d, >34 kg: a single dose of 3 tablets (1.5 g) x 1d, then 2 tablets (1 gram)/d x 6d

—Larval (tissue stage)

Echinococcus granulosus (hydatid cyst)

Drug of choice:	Albendazole[66]	400 mg bid x 28 days, repeated as necessary	15 mg/kg/d x 28 days, repeated as necessary

Echinococcus multilocularis

Treatment of choice:	See footnote [67]		

Cysticercus cellulosae (cysticercosis)

Drug of choice:[68]	Praziquantel[7]	50 mg/kg/d in 3 doses x 15d	50 mg/kg/d in 3 doses x 15d
	OR		
	Albendazole	15 mg/kg/d in 3 doses x 8d, repeated as necessary	15 mg/kg/d in 3 doses x 8d, repeated as necessary
Alternative:	Surgery		

Infection	Drug	Adult Dosage*	Pediatric Dosage*
Toxocariasis, *See* VISCERAL LARVA MIGRANS			

TOXOPLASMOSIS *(Toxoplasma gondii)*[69]

Drugs of choice:	Pyrimethamine[70]	25–100 mg/d x 3–4 wks	2 mg/kg/d x 3d, then 1 mg/kg/d (max. 25 mg/d) x 4 wks[71]
	plus sulfadiazine	1–2 grams qid x 3–4 wks	100–200 mg/kg/d x 3–4 wks
Alternative:	Spiramycin	3–4 grams/d[72]	50–100 mg/kg/d x 3–4 wks

TRICHINOSIS *(Trichinella spiralis)*

Drugs of choice:	Steroids for severe symptoms		
	plus mebendazole[7,73]	200–400 mg tid x 3d, then 400–500 mg tid x 10d	

TRICHOMONIASIS *(Trichomonas vaginalis)*

Drug of choice:[74]	Metronidazole[3]	2 grams once or 250 mg tid orally x 7d	15 mg/kg/d orally in 3 doses x 7d
	OR		
	Tinidazole[4]	2 grams once	50 mg/kg once (max. 2 grams)

TRICHOSTRONGYLUS infection

Drug of choice:	Pyrantel pamoate[7]	11 mg/kg once (max. 1 gram)	11 mg/kg once (max. 1 gram)
Alternative:	Mebendazole[7]	100 mg bid x 3d	100 mg bid x 3d
	OR		
	Albendazole	400 mg once	400 mg once

TRICHURIASIS *(Trichuris trichiura,* whipworm)

Drug of choice:	Mebendazole	100 mg bid x 3d	100 mg bid x 3d
	OR		
	Albendazole	400 mg once[75]	400 mg once[75]

TRYPANOSOMIASIS

T. cruzi **(South American trypanosomiasis, Chagas' disease)**

Drug of choice:	Nifurtimox[2,76]	8–10 mg/kg/d orally in 4 doses x 120d	1–10 yrs: 15–20 mg/kg/d in 4 doses x 90d; 11–16 yrs: 12.5–15 mg/kg/d in 4 doses x 90d
Alternative:	Benznidazole[77]	5–7 mg/kg/d x 30–120d	

Infection	Drug	Adult Dosage*	Pediatric Dosage*
TRYPANOSOMIASIS *(continued)*			

T. brucei gambiense; T. b. rhodesiense (African trypanosomiasis, sleeping sickness)

hemolymphatic stage

Infection	Drug	Adult Dosage*	Pediatric Dosage*
Drug of choice:	Suramin[2]	100–200 mg (test dose) IV, then 1 gram IV on days 1, 3, 7, 14, and 21	20 mg/kg on days 1, 3, 7, 14, and 21
	OR Eflornithine	see footnote 78	
Alternative:	Pentamidine isethionate[7]	4 mg/kg/d IM x 10d	4 mg/kg/d IM x 10d

late disease with CNS involvement

Infection	Drug	Adult Dosage*	Pediatric Dosage*
Drug of choice:	Melarsoprol[2,79]	2–3.6 mg/kg/d IV x 3 doses; after 1 wk 3.6 mg/kg per day IV x 3 doses, repeat again after 10–21 days	18–25 mg/kg total over 1 month; initial dose of 0.36 mg/kg IV, increasing gradually to max. 3.6 mg/kg at intervals of 1–5d for total of 9–10 doses
	OR Eflornithine	see footnote 78	
Alternatives:	Tryparsamide	One injection of 30 mg/kg (max. 2g) IV every 5d to total of 12 injections, may be repeated after 1 month)	
	plus suramin[2]	One injection of 10 mg/kg IV every 5d to total of 12 injections; may be repeated after 1 month	

VISCERAL LARVA MIGRANS[80]

Infection	Drug	Adult Dosage*	Pediatric Dosage*
Drug of choice:[81]	Diethylcarbamazine[7]	6 mg/kg/d in 3 doses x 7–10d	6 mg/kg/d in 3 doses x 7–10d
Alternatives:	Thiabendazole	50 mg/kg/d in 2 doses x 5d (max. 3 grams/d)[11]	50 mg/kg/d in 2 doses x 5d (max. 3 grams/d)[11]
	Mebendazole[7]	100–200 mg bid x 5d[82]	

Whipworm, See TRICHURIASIS

Wuchereria bancrofti, See FILARIASIS

*The letter d stands for day.

1. Dosage and duration of administration should not be exceeded because of possibility of causing optic neuritis; maximum dosage is 2 grams/day.
2. In the USA, this drug is available from the CDC Drug Service, Centers for Disease Control, Atlanta, Georgia 30333; telephone: 404-639-3670 (evenings, weekends, and holidays: 404-639-2888).
3. Metronidazole is carcinogenic in rodents and mutagenic in bacteria; it should generally not be given to pregnant women, particularly in the first trimester.
4. A nitro-imidazole similar to metronidazole, but not marketed in the USA; tinidazole appears to be at least as effective as metronidazole and better tolerated. Ornidazole, a similar drug, is also used outside the USA.
5. Contraindicated in pregnancy.
6. One patient with a *Naegleria* infection was successfully treated with amphotericin B, miconazole, and rifampin (JS Seidel et al, N Engl J Med, 306:346, 1982).
7. An approved drug, but considered investigational for this condition by the U.S. Food and Drug Administration.
8. Strains of *Acanthamoeba* isolated from fatal granulomatous amebic encephalitis are usually sensitive *in vitro* to pentamidine, ketoconazole *(Nizoral)*, 5-fluorocytosine, and (less so) to amphotericin B (RJ Duma et al, Antimicrob Agents Chemother, 10:370, 1976). For treatment of keratitis caused by *Acanthamoeba*, concurrent topical use of 0.1% propamidine isethionate *(Broline*—Rhône-Poulenc Rorer, Canada) plus neosporin, or oral itraconazole *(Sporanox*— Janssen) plus topical miconazole, has been successful (MB Moore and JP McCulley, Br J Ophthalmol, 73:271, 1989; Y Ishibashi et al, Am J Ophthalmol, 109:121, 1990).
9. Effectiveness documented only in animals.
10. Most patients recover spontaneously without antiparasitic drug therapy. Analgesics, corticosteroids, and careful removal of CSF at frequent intervals can relieve symptoms (J. Koo et al, Rev Infect Dis, 10:1155, 1988). Albendazole, levamisole *(Ergamisol)*, or ivermectin has also been used successfully in animals.
11. This dose is likely to be toxic and may have to be decreased.
12. Azithromycin *(Zithromax)* 150 mg/kg plus quinine has been effective in experimental animals. Concurrent use of pentamidine and trimethoprimsulfamethoxazole has been reported to cure an infection with *B. divergens* (D Raoult et al, Ann Intern Med, 107:944, 1987).
13. Not recommended for children less than eight years old.
14. Drugs that could be tried include diethylcarbamazine, levamisole, and fenbendazole (KR Kazacos, J Am Vet Med Assoc, 195:894, 1989) and ivermectin. Steroiod therapy may be helpful, especially in eye or CNS infection. Ocular baylisascariasis has been treated successfully using laser therapy to destroy intraretinal larvae.
15. Clinical significance of these organisms is controversial, but metronidazole 750 mg tid x 10d or iodoquinol 650 mg tid x 20d anecdotally have been reported to be effective (RA Miller and BH Minshew, Rev Infect Dis, 10:930, 1988; PW Doyle et al, J Clin Microbiol, 28:116, 1990).
16. Infection is self-limited in immunocompetent patients. In AIDS patients with large-volume intractable diarrhea, octreotide *(Sandostatin)* 300–500 µg tid subcutaneously may control the diarrhea, but not the infection (DJ Cook et al, Ann Intern Med, 108:708, 1988). Paromomycin may be helpful in some patients (K Clezy et al, AIDS, 5:1146, 1991; J Gathe, Jr et al, Int Conf AIDS, 6:384, 1990).
17. Albendazole 200 mg bid x 3 days has also been reported to be effective (SK Jones et al, Br J Dermatol, 122:99, 1990).
18. Not curative, but decreases inflammation and facilitates removing the worm. Mebendazole 400–800 mg/d for 6d has been reported to kill the worm directly.
19. A single dose of ivermectin, 25–200 µg/kg, has been reported to be effective for treatment of microfilaremia due to *W. bancrofti* and *M. ozzardi* (EA Ottesen et al, N Engl J Med, 322:1113, 1990; M Sabry et al, Trans R Soc Trop Med Hyg, 85:640, 1991; TB Nutman et al, J Infect Dis, 156:662, 1987).
20. Antihistamines or corticosteroids may be required to decrease allergic reactions due to disintegration of microfilariae in treatment of filarial infections, especially those caused by *Loa loa*. Diethylcarbamazine should be administered with special caution in heavy infections with *Loa loa* because it can provoke an encephalopathy (B Carme et al, Am J Trop Med Hyd, 44:684, 1991).

Apheresis has been reported to be effective in lowering microfilarial counts in patients heavily infected with loiasis. Diethylcarbamazine, 300 mg once weekly, has been recommended for prevention of loiasis (TB Nutman et al, N Engl J Med, 319:752, 1988).

21. For patients with no microfilaremia in the blood or skin, full doses can be given from day one.

22. Ivermectin may also be effective.

23. Unlike infections with other flukes, *hepatica* infections may not respond to praziquantel. Limited data, however, indicate that triclabendazole *(Fasinex)*, a veterinary fasciolide, is safe and effective in a single oral dose of 10 mg/kg (L Loutan et al, Lancet, 2:383, 1989).

24. Not absorbed; may be useful for treatment of giardiasis in pregnant women.

25. In sulfonamide-sensitive patients, such as some patients with AIDS, pyrimethamine 50–75 mg daily has been effective (LM Weiss et al, Ann Intern Med, 109:474, 1988). In immunocompromised patients, it may be necessary to continue therapy indefinitely.

26. Limited data indicate that ketoconazole, 400 to 600 mg daily for four to eight weeks, may be effective for treatment of cutaneous and mucosal leishmaniasis (RE Saenz et al, Am J Med, 89:147, 1990).

27. May be repeated or continued. A longer duration may be needed for some forms of visceral leishmaniasis.

28. Recent studies indicate that stibogluconate (pentavalent antimony)-resistant *L. donovani* may respond to recombinant human gamma interferon in addition to antimony (R Badaro et al, N Engl J Med, 322:16, 1990), pentamidine followed by a course of antimony (CP Thakur et al, Am J Trop Med Hyg, 45:435, 1991), or ketoconazole (JP Wali et al, Lancet, 336:810, 1990). Recently, liposomal encapsulated amphotericin B (AmBisome, Vestar, San Dimas, CA) was used successfully to treat multiple-drug-resistant visceral leishmaniasis (RN Davidson et al, Lancet, 337:1061, 1991).

29. Application of heat 39° to 42°C directly to the lesion for 20 to 32 hours over a period of 10 to 12 days has been reported to be effective in cutaneous *L. tropica* (FA Neva et al, Am J Trop Med Hyg, 33:800, 1984).

30. For infestation of eyelashes with crab lice, use petrolatum.

31. FDA-approved only for head lice.

32. Some consultants recommend a second application one week later to kill hatching progeny. Seizures have been reported in association with the use of lindane. Do not use higher than recommended doses and avoid warm baths before application (M Tenenbein, J Am Geriatr Soc, 39:394, 1991). Prolonged use of lindane has been associated with aplastic anemia (AE Rauch et al, Arch Intern Med, 150:2393, 1990.)

33. If chloroquine phosphate is not available, hydroxychloroquine sulfate is as effective; 400 mg of hydroxychloroquine sulfate is equivalent to 500 mg of chloroquine phosphate.

34. In *P. falciparum* malaria, if the patient has not shown a response to conventional doses of chloroquine in 48–72 hours, parasitic resistance to this drug should be considered. *P. vivax* with decreased susceptibility to chloroquine has been reported from Papua New Guinea (KH Rieckmann et al, Lancet, 2:1183, 1989) and from Indonesia (IK Schwartz et al, N Engl J Med, 324:927, 1991). Intramuscular injection of chloroquine can be painful and has been reported to cause abscesses.

35. A recent study found artemether, a Chinese drug, effective for parenteral treatment of severe malaria in children (NJ White et al, Lancet, 339:317, 1992).

36. Some experts consider quinidine more effective than quinine. EKG monitoring is necessary to detect arrhythmias. Oral drugs should be substituted as soon as possible.

37. Not available in the USA. *P. falciparum* infections with a high parasitemia may require a loading dose of 20 mg/kg (NJ White et al, Am J Trop Med Hyg, 32:1, 1983). IV administration of quinine dihydrochloride can be hazardous; constant monitoring of the pulse and blood pressure is necessary to detect arrhythmia or hypotension. Use of parenteral quinine may also lead to severe hypoglycemia; blood glucose should be monitored. Oral drugs should be substituted as soon as possible.

38. Chloroquine-resistant *P. falciparum* infections have been reported in all areas that have malaria except Central America north of Panama, Mexico, Haiti, the Dominican Republic, and the Middle East (including Egypt). In pregnancy, chloroquine prophylaxis has been used extensively and safely, but the safety of other prophylactic antimalarial agents in pregnancy is unclear. Therefore, travel during pregnancy to chloroquine-resistant areas should be discouraged. For chloroquine-

resistant parasitemia > 10%, exchange transfusion has been used (KD Miller et al, N Engl J Med, 321:65, 1989; M Saddler et al; F Vachon et al; KD Miller et al, N Engl J Med, 322:58, 1990).

39. Chloroquine-resistant *falciparum* malaria acquired outside of Southeast Asia, East Africa, Bangladesh, Oceania, and the Amazon basin is likely to respond to quinine (or quinidine) plus pyrimethamine-sulfadoxine. In pregnancy, quinine (or quinidine) plus clindamycin is a reasonable alternative.

40. Although quinine will usually control an attack of resistant *falciparum* malaria, in a substantial number of infections from Southeast Asia, Bangladesh, Oceania, East Africa, and the Amazon region it fails to prevent recurrence. In these regions, there may be pyrimethamine-sulfadoxine resistance, and addition of tetracycline or clindamycin may decrease the rate of recurrence.

41. In Southeast Asia, there is a relative increase in resistance to quinine and the usual treatment dose should be extended to seven days.

42. *Fansidar* tablets contain 25 mg of pyrimethamine and 500 mg of sulfadoxine.

43. At this dosage, adverse effects including nausea, vomiting, diarrhea, dizziness, disturbed sense of balance, toxic psychosis, and seizures can occur. Mefloquine is teratogenic in animals. It should not be given together with quinine or quinidine, and caution is required in using quinine or quinidine to treat patients with malaria who have taken mefloquine for prophylaxis. The pediatric dosage has not been approved by the FDA.

44. In the USA, a 250-mg tablet of mefloquine contains 228 mg of mefloquine base. Outside the USA, each 274-mg tablet contains 250 mg base.

45. Outside the USA, the manufacturer recommends dividing the 1250-mg dose into 750 mg followed 6–8 hours later by 500 mg (D Kingston, Med J Aust, 153:235, 1990).

46. NJ White, Eur J Clin Pharm, 34:1, 1988.

47. May be effective in multiple-drug-resistant *falciparum* malaria (ed., Lancet, 2:537, 1989). Failures in treatment of multiple-drug-resistant malaria have, however, been reported (GD Shanks et al, Am J Trop Med Hyg, 45:488, 1991). For patients with minimal previous exposure to malaria, a second course of therapy is recommended one week after the first course.

48. Primaquine phosphate can cause hemolytic anemia, especially in patients whose red cells are deficient in glucose-6-phosphate dehydrogenase. This deficiency is most common in Blacks, Orientals, and Mediterranean peoples. Patients should be screened for G-6-PD deficiency before treatment. Primaquine should not be used during pregnancy.

49. At present, no drug regimen guarantees protection against malaria. If fever develops within a year (particularly within the first two months) after travel to malarious areas, travelers should be advised to seek medical attention. Insect repellents, insecticide-impregnated bed nets, and proper clothing are important adjuncts for malaria prophylaxis.

50. For prevention of attack after departure from areas where *P. vivax* and *P. ovale* are endemic, which includes almost all areas where malaria is found (except Haiti), some experts in addition prescribe primaquine phosphate 15 mg base (26.3 mg)/d or, for children, 0.3 mg base/kg/d during the last two weeks of prophylaxis. Others prefer to avoid the toxicity of primaquine and rely on surveillance to detect cases when they occur, particularly when exposure was limited or doubtful. See also footnote 48.

51. For prophylaxis where both chloroquine and pyrimethamine/sulfadoxine resistance coexist, mefloquine is the usual drug of choice. In mefloquine-resistant areas, such as Thailand, doxycycline is recommended.

52. The pediatric dosage has not been approved by the FDA, and the drug has not been approved for use during pregnancy. Women should take contraceptive precautions while taking mefloquine and for two months after the last dose. Mefloquine is not recommended for children weighing less than 15 kg, or for patients taking beta-blockers, calcium-channel blockers, or other drugs that may prolong or otherwise alter cardiac conduction. Patients with a history of seizures or psychiatric disorders and those whose occupation requires fine coordination or spatial discrimination should probably avoid mefloquine (Medical Letter, 32:13, 1990).

53. Beginning one week before travel and continuing weekly for the duration of stay and for four weeks after leaving.

54. Beginning one day before travel and continuing for the duration of stay and for four weeks after leaving. The FDA considers use of tetracyclines as antimalarials to be investigational. Use of tetracyclines is contraindicated in pregnancy and in children less than eight years old. Physicians

who prescribe doxycycline as malaria chemoprophylaxis should advise patients to use an appropriate sunscreen (Medical Letter, 31:59, 1989) to minimize the possibility of a photosensitivity reaction and should warn women that *Candida* vaginitis is a frequent adverse effect.

55. Resistance to *Fansidar* should be anticipated in Southeast Asia, Bangladesh, Oceania, the Amazon basin, and in east Africa. Use of *Fansidar* is contraindicated in patients with a history of sulfonamide or pyrimethamine intolerance. In pregnancy at term and in infants less than two months old, pyrimethamine-sulfadoxine may cause hyperbilirubinemia.

56. Proguanil (*Paludrine*—Ayerst, Canada; ICI, England), which is not available in the USA but is widely available overseas, is recommended mainly for use in Africa south of the Sahara. Failures in prophylaxis with chloroquine and proguanil have, however, been reported in travelers to Kenya (AJ Barnes, Lancet, 338:1338, 1991).

57. In a limited number of patients with severe diarrhea, albendazole 400 mg bid for 4–6 weeks was reported to produce remission (C Blanshard et al, Int Conf AIDS, 7:248, 1991). Octreotide (*Sandostatin*, Sandoz) has provided symptomatic relief (JP Cello et al, Ann Intern Med, 115:705, 1991).

58. A keratopathy in an AIDS patient was treated successfully with surgical debridement, topical antibiotics, and itraconazole (*Sporanox*—Janssen) (RW Yee et al, Ophthalmology, 98:196, 1991).

59. AIDS patients should be treated for 21 days. In moderate or severe PCP with room air $PO_2\leq70$ mmHg or Aa gradient ≥35 mmHg prednisone should also be used (Medical Letter, 33:101, 1991).

60. Assay for G-6-PD deficiency recommended at start of therapy.

61. Each double-strength tablet contains 160 mg TMP and 800 mg SMX.

62. Contraindicated in pregnancy. Neuropsychiatric disturbances and seizures have been reported in some patients (H Stokvis et al, Am J Trop Med Hyg, 35:330, 1986).

63. In east Africa, the dose should be increased to 30 mg/kg, and in Egypt and South Africa, 30 mg/kg/d x 2d. Some experts recommend 40–60 mg/kg over 2–3 days in all of Africa (KC Shekhar, Drugs, 42:379, 1991).

64. In immunocompromised patients it may be necessary to continue therapy or use other agents.

65. In disseminated strongyloidiasis, thiabendazole therapy should be continued for at least five days.

66. With a fatty meal to enhance absorption. Some patients may benefit from or require surgical resection of cysts (RK Tompkins, Mayo Clin Proc, 66:1281, 1991). Praziquantel may also be useful preoperatively or in case of spill during surgery.

67. Surgical excision is the only reliable means of treatment, although some reports have suggested use of albendazole or mebendazole (JF Wilson et al, Am J Trop Med Hyg, 37:162, 1987; A Davis et al, Bull WHO, 64:383, 1986).

68. Corticosteroids should be given for two to three days before and during drug therapy. Any cysticercocidal drug may cause irreparable damage when used to treat ocular or spinal cysts, even when corticosteroids are used.

69. In ocular toxoplasmosis, corticosteroids should also be used for anti-inflammatory effect on the eyes.

70. Pyrimethamine is teratogenic in animals. To prevent hematological toxicity from pyrimethamine, it is advisable to give leucovorin (folinic acid), about 10 mg/day, either by injection or orally. Some clinicians use pyrimethamine 50 to 100 mg daily after a loading dose of 200 mg with a sulfonamide to treat CNS toxoplasmosis in patients with AIDS and, when sulfonamide sensitivity developed, have given clindamycin 1.8 to 2.4 g/d in divided doses instead of the sulfonamide. In AIDS patients, chronic suppressive treatment with lower dosage should continue indefinitely (Medical Letter, 34:95, 1991; B Danneman et al, Ann Intern Med, 116:33, Jan 1, 1992).

71. Congenitally infected newborns should be treated with pyrimethamine every two or three days and a sulfonamide daily for about one year (JS Remington and G Desmonts in JS Remington and JO Klein, eds, *Infectious Disease of the Fetus and Newborn Infant*, 3rd ed, Philadelphia: Saunders, 1990, page 89).

72. For treatment during pregnancy, continue the drug until delivery.

73. Albendazole or flubendazole (not available in the USA) may also be effective for this indication.

74. Sexual partners should be treated simultaneously. Outside the USA, ornidazole has also been used for this condition. Metronidazole-resistant strains have been reported; higher doses of metronidazole for longer periods are sometimes effective against these strains (J Lossick, Rev Infect Dis, 12:S665, 1990).

75. In heavy infection it may be necessary to extend therapy for 3 days.
76. The addition of gamma interferon to nifurtimox for 20 days in a limited number of patients and in experimental animals appears to have shortened the acute phase of Chagas' disease (RE McCabe et al, J Infect Dis, 163:912, 1991).
77. Limited data.
78. In *T. b. gambiense* infections, eflornithine is highly effective in both the hemolymphatic and CNS stages. Its effectiveness in *T. b. rhodesiense* infections has been variable. Some clinicians have given 400 mg/kg/d IV in 4 divided doses for 14 days, followed by oral treatment with 300 mg/kg/d for 3–4 weeks (F Doua et al, Am J Trop Med Hyg, 37:525, 1987).
79. In frail patients, begin with as little as 18 mg and increase the dose progressively. Pretreatment with suramin has been advocated for debilitated patients. Corticosteroids have been used to prevent arsenical encephalopathy (J Pepin et al, Lancet, 1:1246, 1989).
80. For severe symptoms or eye involvement, corticosteroids can be used in addition.
81. Ivermectin or albendazole may also be effective (D Stürchler et al, Ann Trop Med Parasitol, 83:473, 1989).
82. One report of a cure using 1 gram tid for 21 days has been published (A Bekhti, Ann Intern Med, 100:463, 1984).

ADVERSE EFFECTS OF SOME ANTIPARASITIC DRUGS*

ALBENDAZOLE (*Zentel*)
Occasional: diarrhea; abdominal pain; migration of *ascaris* through mouth and nose
Rare: leukopenia; alopecia; increased serum transaminase activity

BENZNIDAZOLE (*Rochagan*)
Frequent: allergic rash; dose-dependent polyneuropathy; gastrointestinal disturbances; psychic disturbances

BITHIONOL (*Bitin*)
Frequent: photosensitivity reactions; vomiting; diarrhea; abdominal pain; urticaria
Rare: leukopenia; toxic hepatitis

CHLOROQUINE HCl and CHLOROQUINE PHOSPHATE (*Aralen*, and others)
Occasional: pruritis; vomiting; headache; confusion; depigmentation of hair; skin eruptions; corneal opacity; weight loss; partial alopecia; extraocular muscle palsies; exacerbation of psoriasis, eczema, and other exfoliative dermatoses; myalgias; photophobia
Rare: irreversible retinal injury (especially when total dosage exceeds 100 grams); discoloration of nails and mucus membranes; nerve-type deafness; peripheral neuropathy and myopathy; heart block; blood dyscrasias; hematemesis

CROTAMITON (*Eurax*)
Occasional: rash; conjunctivitis

DEHYDROEMETINE
Frequent: cardiac arrhythmias; precordial pain; muscle weakness; cellulitis at site of injection
Occasional: diarrhea; vomiting; peripheral neuropathy; heart failure; headache; dyspnea

DIETHYLCARBAMAZINE CITRATE USP (*Hetrazan*)
Frequent: severe allergic or febrile reactions in patients with microfilaria in the blood or the skin; GI disturbances
Rare: encephalopathy

*Drug interactions are generally not included here; see the current edition of *The Medical Letter Handbook of Adverse Drug Interactions.*

DILOXANIDE FUROATE *(Furamide)*
Frequent: flatulence
Occasional: nausea; vomiting; diarrhea
Rare: diplopia; dizziness; urticaria; pruritus

EFLORNITHINE (Difluoromethylornithine, DFMO, *Ornidyl*)
Frequent: anemia; leukopenia
Occasional: diarrhea; thrombocytopenia; seizures
Rare: hearing loss

FLUBENDAZOLE—similar to mebendazole

FURAZOLIDONE *(Furoxone)*
Frequent: nausea; vomiting
Occasional: allergic reactions, including pulmonary infiltration, hypotension, urticaria, fever, vesicular rash; hypoglycemia; headache
Rare: hemolytic anemia in G-6-PD deficiency and neonates; disulfiram-like reaction with alcohol; MAO-inhibitor interactions; polyneuritis

HALOFANTRINE *(Halfan)*
Occasional: diarrhea; abdominal pain; pruritus

IODOQUINOL *(Yodoxin)*
Occasional: rash; acne; slight enlargement of the thyroid gland; nausea; diarrhea; cramps; anal pruritus
Rare: optic atrophy, loss of vision, peripheral neuropathy after prolonged use in high dosage (for months); iodine sensitivity

IVERMECTIN *(Mectizan)*
Occasional: Mazzotti-type reaction seen in onchocerciasis, including fever, pruritus, tender lymph nodes, headache, and joint and bone pain
Rare: hypotension

LINDANE *(Kwell;* and others)
Occasional: eczematous rash; conjunctivitis
Rare: convulsions; aplastic anemia

MALATHION *(Ovide)*
Occasional: local irritation

MEBENDAZOLE *(Vermox)*
Occasional: diarrhea; abdominal pain; migration of *ascaris* through mouth and nose
Rare: leukopenia; agranulocytosis; hypospermia

MEFLOQUINE *(Lariam)*
Frequent: vertigo; lightheadedness; nausea; other gastrointestinal disturbances; nightmares; visual disturbances; headache
Occasional: confusion
Rare: psychosis; hypotension; convulsions; coma

MEGLUMINE ANTIMONIATE *(Glucantime)* Similar to stibogluconate sodium

MELARSOPROL *(Arsobal)*
Frequent: myocardial damage; albuminuria; hypertension; colic; Herxheimer-type reaction; encephalopathy; vomiting; peripheral neuropathy
Rare: shock

METRONIDAZOLE *(Flagyl,* and others)
Frequent: nausea; headache; dry mouth; metallic taste
Occasional: vomiting; diarrhea; insomnia; weakness; stomatitis; vertigo; paresthesias; rash; dark urine; urethral burning; disulfiram-like reaction with alcohol
Rare: seizures; encephalopathy; pseudomembranous colitis; ataxia; leukopenia; peripheral neuropathy; pancreatitis

NICLOSAMIDE *(Niclocide)*
Occasional: nausea; abdominal pain

NIFURTIMOX *(Lampit)*
Frequent: anorexia; vomiting; weight loss; loss of memory; sleep disorders; tremor; paresthesias; weakness; polyneuritis
Rare: convulsions; fever; pulmonary infiltrates and pleural effusion

ORNIDAZOLE *(Tiberal)*
Occasional: dizziness; headache; gastrointestinal disturbances
Rare: reversible peripheral neuropathy

OXAMNIQUINE *(Vansil)*
Occasional: headache; fever; dizziness; somnolence; nausea; diarrhea; rash; insomnia; hepatic enzyme changes; ECG changes; EEG changes; orange-red discoloration of urine
Rare: seizures; neuropsychiatric disturbances

PAROMOMYCIN *(Humatin)*
Frequent: GI disturbances
Rare: eighth-nerve damage (mainly auditory); renal damage

PENTAMIDINE ISETHIONATE *(Pentam 300, NebuPent)*
Frequent: hypotension; hypoglycemia often followed by diabetes mellitus; vomiting; blood dyscrasias; renal damage; pain at injection site; GI disturbances
Occasional: may aggravate diabetes; shock; hypocalcemia; liver damage; cardiotoxicity; delirium; rash
Rare: Herxheimer-type reaction; anaphylaxis; acute pancreatitis; hyperkalemia

PERMETHRIN *(Nix, Elimite)*
Occasional: burning; stinging; numbness; increased pruritus; pain; edema; erythema; rash

PRAZIQUANTEL *(Biltricide)*
Frequent: malaise; headache; dizziness
Occasional: sedation; abdominal discomfort; fever; sweating; nausea; eosinophilia; fatigue
Rare: pruritus; rash

PRIMAQUINE PHOSPHATE USP
Frequent: hemolytic anemia in G-6-PD deficiency
Occasional: neutropenia; GI disturbances; methemoglobinemia in G-6-PD deficiency

Rare: CNS symptoms; hypertension; arrhythmias

PROGUANIL *(Paludrine)*
Occasional: oral ulceration; hair loss; scaling of palms and soles
Rare: hematuria (with large doses); vomiting; abdominal pain; diarrhea (with large doses)

PYRANTEL PAMOATE *(Antiminth)*
Occasional: GI disturbances; headache; dizziness; rash; fever

PYRETHRINS and PIPERONYL BUTOXIDE (*RID*, others)
Occasional: allergic reactions

PYRIMETHAMINE USP *(Daraprim)*
Occasional: blood dyscrasias; folic acid deficiency
Rare: rash; vomiting; convulsions; shock; possibly pulmonary eosinophilia

QUINACRINE HCl USP *(Atabrine)*
Frequent: dizziness; headache; vomiting; diarrhea
Occasional: yellow staining of skin; toxic psychosis; insomnia; bizarre dreams; blood dyscrasias; urticaria; blue and black nail pigmentation; psoriasis-like rash
Rare: acute hepatic necrosis; convulsions; severe exfoliative dermatitis; ocular effects similar to those caused by chloroquine

QUININE DIHYDROCHLORIDE and SULFATE
Frequent: cinchonism (tinnitus, headache, nausea, abdominal pain, visual disturbance)
Occasional: deafness; hemolytic anemia; other blood dyscrasias; photosensitivity reactions; hypoglycemia; arrhythmias; hypotension; drug fever
Rare: blindness; sudden death if injected too rapidly

SPIRAMYCIN *(Rovamycine)*
Occasional: GI disturbances
Rare: allergic reactions

STIBOGLUCONATE SODIUM *(Pentostam)*
Frequent: muscle pain and joint stiffness; nausea; transaminase elevations; T-wave flattening or inversion
Occasional: weakness; colic; liver damage; bradycardia; leukopenia
Rare: diarrhea; rash; pruritus; myocardial damage; hemolytic anemia; renal damage; shock; sudden death

SURAMIN SODIUM *(Germanin)*
Frequent: vomiting; pruritus; urticaria; paresthesias; hyperesthesia of hands and feet; photophobia; peripheral neuropathy
Occasional: kidney damage; blood dyscrasias; shock; optic atrophy

THIABENDAZOLE *(Mintezol)*
Frequent: nausea; vomiting; vertigo
Occasional: leukopenia; crystalluria; rash; hallucinations; olfactory disturbance; erythema multiforme; Stevens-Johnson syndrome
Rare: shock; tinnitus; intrahepatic cholestasis; convulsions; angioneurotic edema

TINIDAZOLE *(Fasigyn)*
Occasional: metallic taste; nausea; vomiting; rash

TRIMETREXATE (with "leucovorin rescue")
Occasional: rash; peripheral neuropathy; bone marrow depression; increased serum aminotransferase concentrations

TRYPARSAMIDE
Frequent: nausea; vomiting
Occasional: impaired vision; optic atrophy; fever; exfoliative dermatitis; allergic reactions; tinnitus

Reprinted with permission from *The Medical Letter on Drugs and Therapeutics*, Vol. 34 (Issue 865), March 6, 1992, pps. 17–26.

Index

Parasites
  classification of, 37
  definition of, 21
Parasitic Disease Consultants
  Laboratory, 102
Parasitism, 22
Parasitology, 8, 141
Parasitology Laboratory of
  Washington, Inc., 102
Parcells, Hazell, D.C., N.D.,
  Ph.D., 2, 7, 67
Parrish, Louis, M.D., 2, 9, 93,
  117
Perforation, 35, 55
Pennsylvania, 59
Pets, 10, 15–16, 68, 69–77, 80,
  88, 124, 125, 133–136
  questionnaire regarding, 82–
  83
Pig, 48, 63
Pinworms, 3, 18, 22, 24, 37, 47,
  79, 88, 93
  preventing, 124, 133
  symptoms of, 47, 86, 87
  testing for, 97, 98, 136
  treatment of, 104, 107, 113,
  116, 166, 172
Plasmodium falciparum, 28, 44
Plasmodium malariae, 28, 44
Plasmodium ovale, 28, 44
Plasmodium vivax, 28, 44
Platyhelminthes, 26–28
Pneumocystis carinii, 18, 30,
  43–44
  symptoms of, 31, 43–44
  testing for, 98, 99
  treatment of, 172–173
Pneumonia, 30
  symptoms of, 31
Proglottid, 52, 53
Prostaglandin, 23
Protein, 110–111
Protozoa, 23, 28–31, 37, 38–
  45

Questionnaire, 80–85, 86, 91

Racoons, 136
Refugee. *See* Immigrants.
Restaurants, 14, 16, 131, 135
Rhode Island, 44
Risk factors, 9–19
Rivers, 58
Rochlitz, Steven, Ph.D., 12
Rodents, 63, 136
Roundworms, 3, 11, 16, 22,
  24–26, 37, 45–46, 70, 71, 79,
  87, 109, 111, 113, 134
  preventing, 136
  symptoms of, 11, 46, 72, 134
  testing for, 95, 97, 98, 136
  treatment of, 104, 111, 115,
  116
Russia, 11, 12, 53

Salt, 131
San Diego, 44, 80, 86
San Francisco, 18, 59
Sashimi, 16, 65, 130
Scandinavia, 53
Schistosoma haematobium, 28
Schistosoma japonicum, 28, 54
Schistosoma mansoni, 26, 54
Schistosomes, 22
Schistosomiasis, 8, 28, 54, 88, 89
  treatment of, 105, 173
Scolex, 51
Seafood, 130
Seatworm, 24
Sexual practices, 132–133
  questionnaire regarding, 83
Sexual revolution, 10, 17–18
Silverware, 67
"60 Minutes," 70
Sleeping sickness, 173
Snails, 54, 89
South America, 10, 14, 44, 54,
  55
South Pacific, 14, 50
Soy products, 111–112
Spores, 43
Stomach acid. *See*
  Hydrochloric acid.